A Caregiver's Complete Guide for Safe Mobility
and Independence in the Home

A Caregiver's Complete Guide for Safe Mobility and Independence in the Home

Kevin F. Lockette, PT

Two Harbors Press

Two Harbors Press
212 3ʳᵈ Avenue North, Suite 290
Minneapolis, MN 55401
612.455.2293
www.TwoHarborsPress.com

NOTE: Physical disability can vary greatly from one person to the next. Health and
wellness require individual consideration. Readers should consult their physicians,
occupational and physical therapists regarding their individual needs with regard to
mobility. This book is not intended to replace professional medical rehabilitation
programs. It should be used as a guide to promote safety in conjunction with the
medical profession. Any application of the recommendations set forth in this book
is at the reader's discretion and risk.

ISBN-13: 978-1-936401-12-3
LCCN: 2010940621

Distributed by Itasca Books

Typeset by Nate Meyers

Printed in the United States of America

This book is dedicated to the memory of Pearl Atkins and to all care-givers who give so much of themselves to help others.

CONTENTS

PREFACE

I have accumulated, during more than 20 years as a physical therapist, a wealth of knowledge, strategies, and tips to make caregiving easier and safer, especially as it relates to mobility and independence. You, as caregivers, must understand a wide spectrum of issues and are faced with daily challenges.

This book is intended to make life for you, the caregiver, a bit easier. If a caregiver is injured, it frequently results in the care-receiver losing the ability to remain in a community setting. The following pages are filled with pragmatic information to assist you in all aspects of caregiving, including assisting with bed mobility and transfers, simple home adaptations, wheelchair selection, adaptive equipment, assisting with exercises, and much more. Included are golden nuggets of knowledge from many perspectives, including from residential and professional caregiving, physical therapy, and occupational therapy.

ACKNOWLEDGEMENTS

This project could not be what it is without the assistance of many. Thank you so much for your contributions.

PARTICIPANTS: Jack Richardson, Lorraine Kent, David Lerps, Ginger Lockette, Kimi Kaneshiro, Debbie Ritchie, Doug Smoyer

EQUIPMENT: All medical equipment for this project was provided by Hawaiian Island Medical (http://www.himed.cc)

PHOTOGRAPHY: Melissa Hinkley

ILLUSTRATIONS: Tiki Wolf (www.face-nook.com)

CONTENT REVIEWERS: Arlene A. Schmid, PhD, OTR; Ginger Lockette, PT; Bruce Katsura, MD; Stanley Bergstrom; Staff of Ohana Pacific Rehab Services, LLC

CHAPTER ONE:

BODY MECHANICS

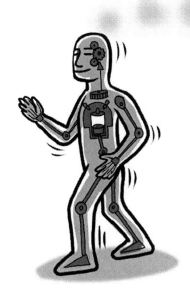

Oh, My Aching Back!

Most back injuries result from poor body mechanics. Poor body mechanics can occur while sitting, standing, working in the yard, and yes, assisting a care-receiver with transfers from the bed to a chair. That ache or fullness in the low back at the end of the day is due to stress on spinal discs, facet joints (where two vertebra connect), muscles, and ligaments. I call these "micro-traumas," and over time, they can add up to produce a full-blown back injury.

Anatomy

The vertebrae (back bones) have two functional areas. The first area is the vertebral body, which is designed and responsible for weight-bearing. This is the area where loading or stress through the spine should take place. The vertebral bodies are separated by sponge-like discs to assist in shock absorption and weight-bearing. The second area is called the facet joint, which is where the vertebrae articulate (connect). The facet joint is responsible for movement and is non-weight-bearing. Poor posture can affect where stress takes place and can cause injury. The low back is the lumbar spine; the middle back is the thoracic spine; and the neck area is the cervical spine. There are normal curves in each of these areas. The normal spinal curves include a gentle low back (lumbar) curve; a gentle, rounded upper back (thoracic); and another gentle curve in the neck (cervical). Maintaining these normal curves minimizes stresses to the back (ligaments, discs, nerves, etc.) and helps to avoid injury.

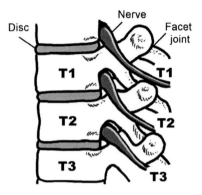

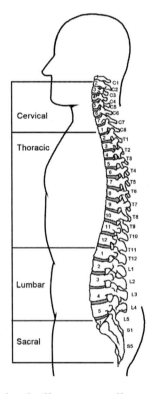

Posture

Good posture is essential for a healthy spine. By maintaining the normal curves mentioned above, the vertebrae are mechanically stacked, which minimizes or eliminates abnormal stresses. Once out of this ideal alignment, stresses occur to the different structures in the neck and back, which ultimately can lead to pain and injury. The three basic types of postures are swayback/excessive curve, flat back, and neutral spine/normal back.

The swayback posture has an excessive lumbar curve and is common in people who have weak abdominals and excessive abdominal fat (pot belly). This excessive curve can lead to mechanical pain and arthritis in the spine by placing stress on the facet joints, which are designed for movement and not weight-bearing.

A flat back is basically a rounded low back, which causes the loss of lumbar (low back) curve. This posture, especially when lifting objects or when transferring care-receivers, can lead to muscular injury or involvement of the intravertebral discs.

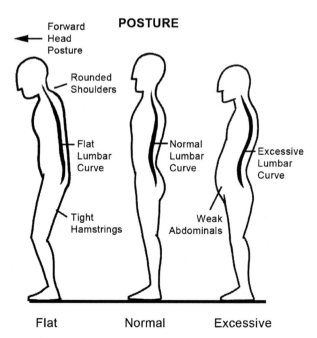

3

Good Body Mechanics

Caregiving, by its very nature, can cause great physical stress on you as the caregiver. Practicing proper body mechanics will decrease the stress and strain and help to safely manage the mobility of the care-receiver. The primary rule is to maintain the normal lumbar curve at *all times*. By following this one simple rule, injury to the lower back can be avoided. This means that you may need to get in different positions or use different transfer techniques, based on your own body type/size and that of the care-receiver. The following lifting principles will help keep the normal lumbar curve.

Principles of Safe Lifting
1. *Maintain a sturdy or broad base of support.* A stable position is necessary when assisting the care-receiver with moving. A wide base of support is stable—spread the feet at or greater than shoulder-width apart—but keep in mind that having the feet in a scissor position, with one foot forward and one foot backward, also offers a wide base of support. The physical space available will dictate which position to use when assisting with moving. For an example, when assisting someone with a car transfer, there may not be enough room to spread the feet shoulder-width apart; therefore, the scissor position may be the better option.

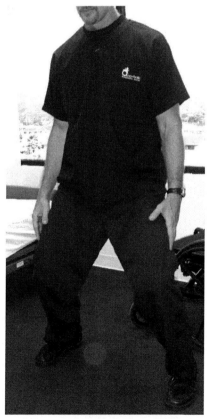 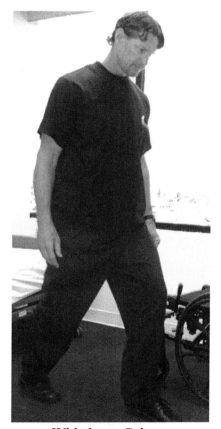

Wide base: Shoulder width   Wide base: Scissor

2. *Keep the load close*. This applies to lifting objects as well as to assisting a care-receiver with a transfer. For example, when lifting a chair, if the chair back is close to the body, it feels much lighter than if the chair is lifted with the arms extended and away from the body. With the latter technique, a strain will be felt in the low back. The farther away the object (or care-receiver) being lifted, the greater the lever arm, which makes the care-receiver or object feel heavier. It is much easier to lift and much easier to keep that normal lumbar curve when the load is closer.

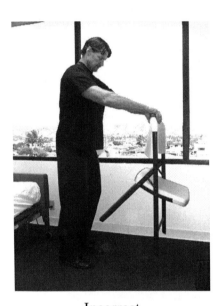 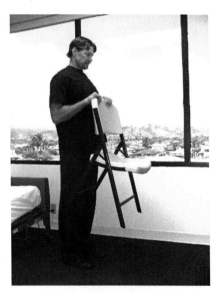

Incorrect   Correct

3. *Bend with the knees, not with the back.* The take-home message here is that bending forward with a rounded low back (lumbar spine) loses the normal lumbar curve and causes stress to your low back. The larger, stronger leg muscles are better equipped to do the lifting than the low-back muscles. Remember to tighten up the stomach and bend down with your legs.

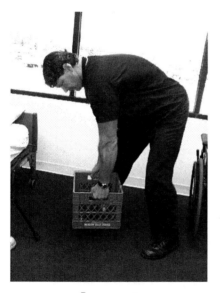 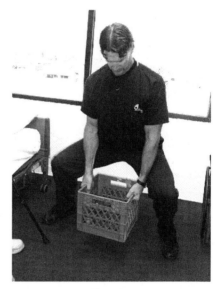

Incorrect   Correct

4. *Push instead of pull, whenever possible.* When pulling a load, it is much harder to keep the normal lumbar curve (neutral spine), so whenever possible, push rather than pull. For example, in assisting a care-receiver up from a low chair, it is better to stand on the side of the care-receiver and push him forward so that his center of gravity is over his feet—so that he can use his legs to transfer to standing—rather than standing in front of him and pulling forward where you are performing more work and potentially placing more strain on your lower back.

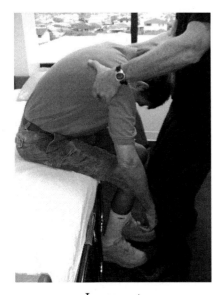

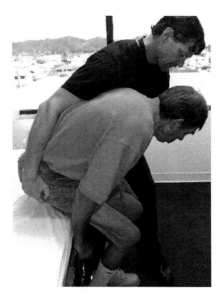

Incorrect	Correct

CHAPTER TWO:

GENERAL MOBILITY GUIDELINES FOR TRANSFERS

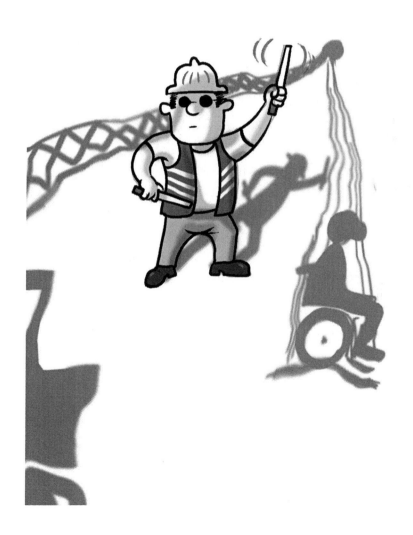

Now that a background for good posture and body mechanics has been established, it is time to apply it when working with care-receivers. The following guidelines will assist in maintaining a normal lumbar curve (neutral spine) and ultimately avoid injury.

Body Positions and Hand Placement, Considering Body Types

Tall or short, small or large, you need to apply the principles of good body mechanics when assisting care-receivers with mobility, although there are differences in how to accomplish this. For example, when a tall person with long arms performs a dependent transfer (requires maximum assist from the caregiver) of an average-sized person, a common approach would be to bend the care-receiver forward and to reach over the care-receiver for hand placement on his hips or transfer belt, as this is the easiest way to keep the care-receiver close to your body, to keep the normal lumbar curve, and to have a stable base of support (see Figure 2.1). If a tall caregiver approached this transfer by positioning himself in front of the care-receiver, with hand placement under the care-receiver's arms, he would have to bend down really low to keep the normal lumbar curve, which is hard on the knees and not as stable a base of support. In contrast, a caregiver of smaller stature most likely would be unable to perform the reaching-over style transfer, as his arms probably would not be long enough to reach over and around the care-receiver. Instead, he might position himself in front of the care-receiver and reach his arms under the care-receiver's arms to keep a neutral spine (Figure 2.2). Any time that the lower back is flat or rounded while lifting, stress will occur to this area, which can result in a back injury. The bottom line is that you must always keep the normal lumbar curve when lifting to avoid injury. You will have to figure out how to position your body and where to place your hands while maintaining the normal lumbar curve (neutral spine). There is no perfect way to do this; it depends on each circumstance. The body type of both the caregiver and care-receiver will dictate which position and hand placement is best.

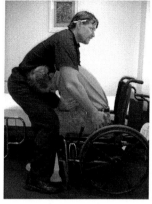 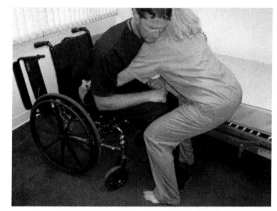

Figure 2.1 Reaching over   Figure 2.2 Reaching under

Considering the Care-Receiver's Assets and Deficits
When assisting a care-receiver with mobility, an important goal should be for the caregiver to perform the least amount of work possible, and for the care-receiver to perform the most amount of work possible. The more the care-receiver participates in his or her own mobility, the more therapeutic it will be for him or her—and the less stress there will be on you as the caregiver. To achieve this, it is important to know the care-receiver's capabilities by understanding his or her physical assets and deficits. For example, can the care-receiver weight-bear through his legs? The more leg strength the care-receiver has, the more he can assist in his own mobility. The amount of strength the care-receiver has will dictate which type of transfer will be the safest. For example, if he is able to weight-bear almost 100 percent by basically standing with his own leg strength, then he most likely will require only spotting/touch assist for balance. If he can weight-bear only 50 percent or less and requires assistance to hold his own body weight when attempting to stand,

then a completely different transfer technique is required. The chart below lists some considerations when assisting the care-receiver.

ASSETS	DEFICITS
Good leg strength and able to weight-bear through legs, once standing Consideration: He may need help with balance but most likely will not require physical assist to hold up his body.	*Poor leg strength, with difficulty bearing weight through legs* Consideration: He will need more physical assistance; possibly not a standing pivot transfer but rather a squat pivot transfer, or a more dependent transfer.
Good cognition Consideration: Can follow transfer commands.	*Has a weak side, such as seen with hemiparesis following a stroke* Consideration: Transfer on stronger side, when possible.
	Dementia Consideration: May not be able to follow transfer commands. May grab during transfers.

Hand Placement for Transfers

Hand placement is an important consideration when assisting a care-receiver with transfers. It's also important to communicate to him where he will be touched, especially for the first time with a transfer. If the care-receiver is unable to weight-bear fully, you, as the care-giver, may need to hold on to his hips. Do not grab his clothes—that is not stable or sturdy, and it also is uncomfortable for the care-receiver, especially if you take hold of the back of the pants. It is better to use a transfer belt or to cup your hands around each side of the care-receiver's buttocks.

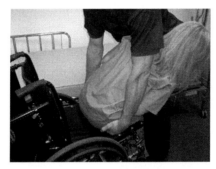

Hand position for transfers: Cup hips

If your arms are not long enough to cup the care-receiver's hips, work a sheet or bath towel underneath the care-receiver's buttocks and hold on to the towel or sheet. This creates an extension and still allows for good control.

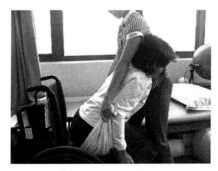

Towel/sheet extension

Considerations for Different Disabilities

- *Parkinson's disease (PD).* PD is a movement disorder that is characterized by stiffness or rigidity in the muscles and difficulty with initiating or terminating movement. One of the primary challenges in assisting with a transfer of someone with PD is the care-receiver's trunk rigidity and lack of power for movements, such as sit-to-stand, as he cannot move very fast. When transferring a person with PD, it is helpful to assist him in bending forward at the hip so he can move from sitting to standing or be able to bear weight through his legs for a squat pivot or standing pivot transfer. Place the care-receiver forward so that his weight is over his feet; then he can assist with the motion of coming to standing (nose past the toes). Rocking forward and back uses momentum that can aid in initiating the movement. Count to three, while rocking the care-receiver forward with each count, to create momentum forward.

- *Total hip replacement.* Someone who has had recent total hip replacement will not be able to cross the leg past the midline of the body, flex/bend her hip past 90 degrees, or rotate her hip inward (toes of replacement side pointing towards opposite leg). These movements are referred to as "total hip precautions." These motions can actually dislocate the hip, so it is important to adhere to these movement restrictions (total hip precautions) with all of the care-receiver's mobility.

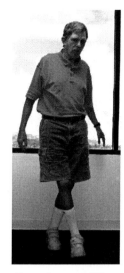 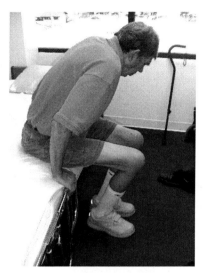 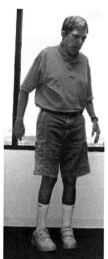

Crossing midline   Bending past 90 degrees   Pointing toes in

In total hip precautions with bed mobility such as rolling or coming to sitting from lying down, put a pillow in between the legs to prevent the leg from crossing midline. With sitting to standing, make sure that the care-receiver keeps the total hip replacement leg straight as he bends forward and that he does not bend the leg past 90 degrees.   To perform sitting to standing, the care-receiver needs to be flexed forward at the hip (nose over toes), which is hip flexion greater than 90 degrees. Anytime that the knee is higher or past the hip, you are greater than 90 degrees. By having the care-receiver straighten his leg on the hip replacement side, the hip angle is less than 90 degrees on the involved side and the care-receiver can still bend forward to assist in coming to standing (see illustrations on page 16).

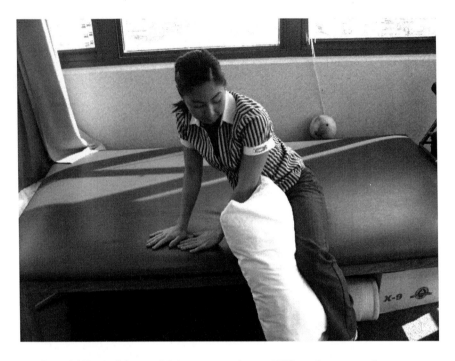

Bed mobility with total hip precautions: Pillow between knees

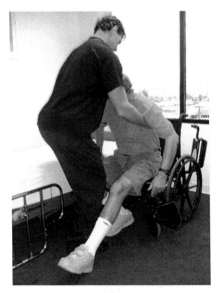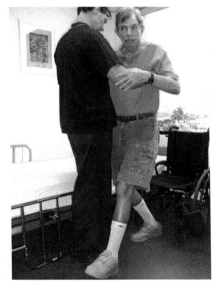

Sit to standing with total hip precautions

- *Stroke with hemiparesis.* Hemiparesis means that one side of the body was affected by the stroke. There is great variability in the degree of disability with hemiparesis. Regardless of the extent of disability, however, it is best to transfer by leading with the care-receiver's strong side, when possible. Some care-receivers will be able to bear weight on their affected side, while others may not. Also, some care-receivers with left hemiparesis may experience "left neglect," a condition in which the person is not aware of the left side. This is a sensory deficit rather than a motor deficit, but it can be challenging for the caregiver to assist with the affected leg when the care-receiver cannot feel it. Help a care-receiver compensate by telling her to turn her head to scan to the left with her right eye. This may allow her to better assist in the transfer.

  For bed mobility such as rolling and getting up from lying down, when possible, the care-receiver can assist more if the strong side is the bottom arm when pushing up from side lying to sitting position in bed.

- *Dementia.* This population is one of the most difficult to assist. It is critical that you protect yourself from injury when transferring a care-receiver with dementia. Generally speaking, such care-receivers fall into one of two categories: "grabber" or "pusher." A grabber will grab the caregiver around the waist or neck and will not let go, but the care-receiver also has a tendency to pull you forward so that you are left off balance and have difficulty in keeping the normal lumbar curve (neutral spine). A pusher tends to straighten out her arms on the side to which you are attempting to transfer and to push away from the direction in which she is heading. When working with pushers and grabbers, you, as the caregiver, will need to get the care-receiver's body as close as possible to your body. Instead of allowing the care-receiver to put his or her arms around your waist or neck, it is better to tuck the care-receiver's arms between your body and his, so that his arms do not interfere with the transfer by either pushing or grabbing.

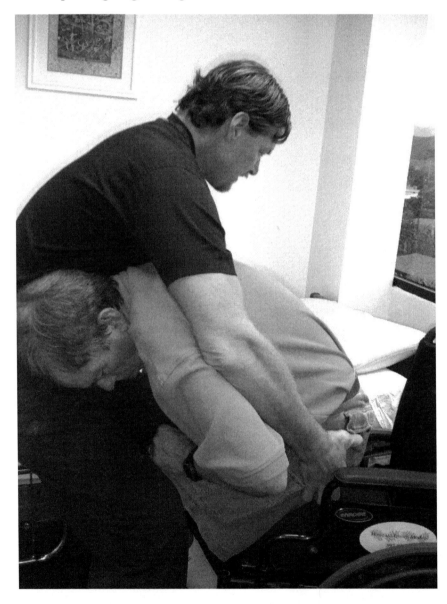

CHAPTER THREE:

BED MOBILITY

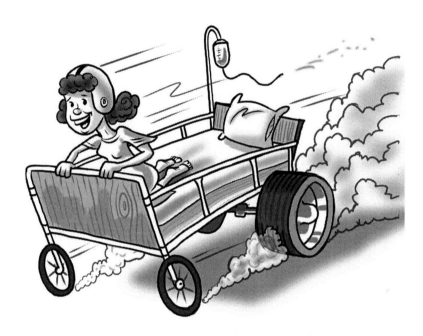

Bed mobility is one activity that can cause repetitive strain on your lower back if not done correctly. It is important to apply good body mechanics and to use techniques that offer you the best advantage. It is all too common to see a caregiver bend forward with a rounded back in an attempt to hoist a care-receiver up to a seated position from lying down. Ultimately, this leads to low back pain and injury to the caregiver's back.

Rolling

The care-receiver typically will be lying on her side, curled in the fetal position; on her back; or on her stomach. If the care-receiver is in the fetal position, you can assist her with rolling by leading with her knees. Keep her knees bent, which gives leverage for rolling. If she is lying flat on her back, bend her knees in a "hook-lying position," in which the knees are bent and the feet are flat on the bed.

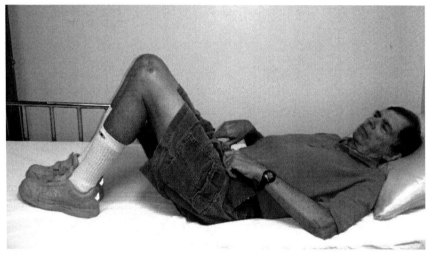

Hook-lying position

If she is lying flat on her stomach, you can "log roll" her by placing your hands on her hip and shoulder and then rolling her until she is lying flat on her back. This technique places little or no stress on your lower back and places her in a position that she will need to be in to transfer from lying to a seated position with her feet off the bed.

Scooting in Bed

There are two options for scooting a care-receiver in bed. If the care-receiver is able to assist, begin in the hook-lying position (lying flat on the back with knees bent and feet flat on the bed) and have the care-receiver perform a "bridge" by lifting his buttocks off the bed. When he lifts his buttocks (forms the bridge), you can then shift his hips in the desired direction. Repeat this until the care-receiver is in the desired position in the bed. This technique works because when the care-receiver lifts his buttocks, movement is easy since there is no friction from the bed and the hips are unweighted.

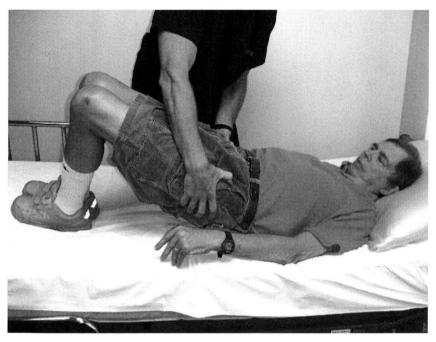

Scooting in bed with bridging

If the care-receiver is dependent (cannot help you/requires maximum assitance), then a draw sheet works best. A draw sheet is a bed sheet that is used to pull the care-receiver to adjust his position in bed. To place a draw sheet, position the care-receiver on his side. Stuff half the sheet under the care-receiver and squish it as far as you can underneath the care-receiver from his back side. Then roll him to the other side and pull the draw sheet through until the sheet is completely under the care-receiver.

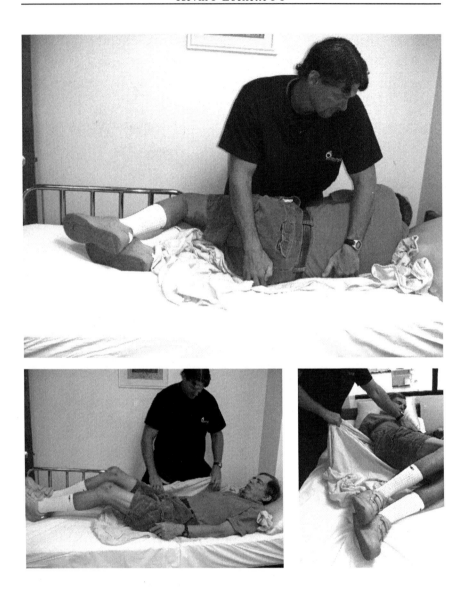

When pulling the draw sheet to reposition the care-receiver, remember to use good body mechanics, even if that means you must put one knee in the bed to keep the normal lumbar curve (neutral spine).

Lying to Sitting

With the lying-to-sitting transfer, most caregivers typically do too much of the work involved and may lose the normal lumbar curve by bending forward to pull the care-receiver up from the bed. This, however, places you in a rounded-back position and can lead to micro-traumas. To avoid placing yourself in this rounded-back position, get the care-receiver in the hook-lying position (knees bent with feet flat on bed), and from there, roll her into a side-lying position. From the side-lying position, slide the care-receiver's legs off the bed. This position will start to pull up the upper trunk. In most circumstances, all that is required to get her into a sitting position is for you to perform a little tug on the pelvis with one hand and a tug on the shoulder with the other hand. This allows the care-receiver the time and ability to get her bottom arm in a position to push all the way to sitting. If the care-receiver has a hard time pushing up, place your hand on her bottom shoulder (the shoulder against the bed) to assist.

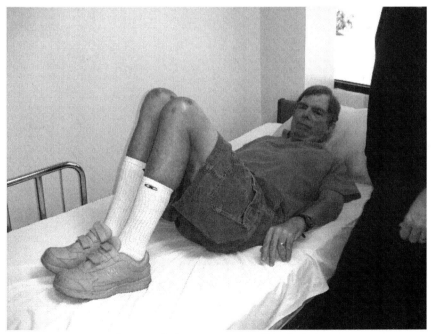

Lying to sitting, step one: Hook-lying

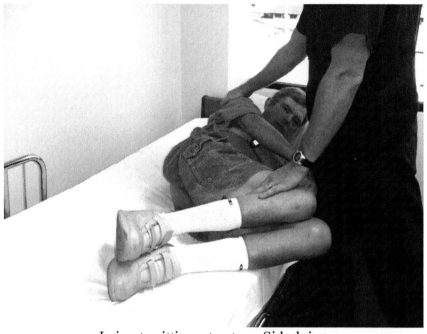

Lying to sitting, step two: Side-lying

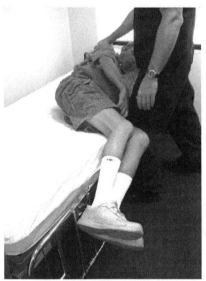

Step three: Legs off bed

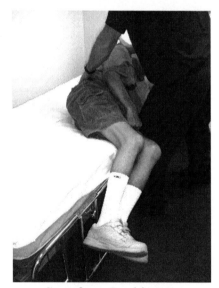

Step four: Pushing up

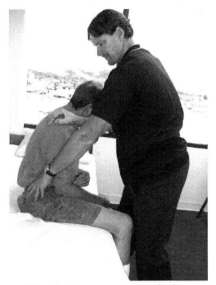 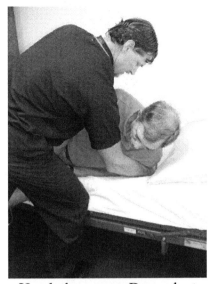

Hand placement: Assisting   Hand placement: Dependent
care-receiver

Hospital Beds

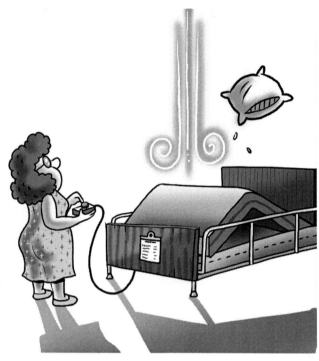

Hospital beds will allow for added flexibility with bed mobility, as the head of the bed can be raised or lowered to assist with the optimal positioning for the transfers. The amount of time and energy you save when the care-receiver is in a hospital bed versus his being in a regular bed depends on the type of hospital bed used. Manual hospital beds typically have a crank system to raise or lower the head of the bed. The crank is usually low to the ground, and it does take some elbow grease to get the head of the bed in the appropriate position. Sometimes, the effort required to crank the bed is greater than just performing the transfer itself. (If you are a small-stature caregiver, however, and your care-receiver is large, this maneuver is worth the effort.) The situation is greatly improved if the care-receiver has an electric bed—a push of the button is all it takes to move the care-receiver up higher or closer to the desired position.

CHAPTER FOUR:

TRANSFERS

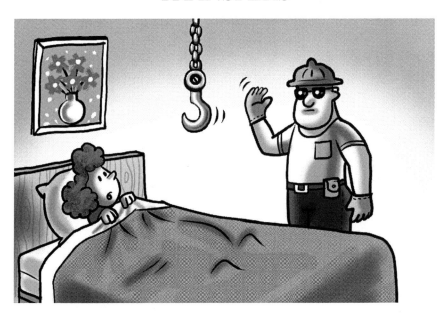

Transfer Preparation

The strategy of transfer preparation is to "stack the cards" in favor of you by setting up things to make the transfer as easy as possible—that is, as the caregiver, you will manipulate the environment as much as possible to your advantage. This can include the position of the chair (or wheelchair), the height of the surface to which (or from which) you are transferring, the stability of the surfaces, and removing any obstacles. Here are a few suggestions:

- *Prepare wheelchair.* Angle the wheelchair close to the surface to which you are transferring the care-receiver. Lock the brakes. If possible, remove the arm rest on the side that is facing the surface to which the care-receiver is transfer-ring. Swing away or remove the leg rest on that same side as well.

- *Bed*. If the bed is a hospital bed, lower or raise the bed to the same level as the chair.
- *Footwear*. Make sure the care-receiver is wearing non-skid footwear. Wearing only socks is a hazard, as they are slippery.

Sit-to-Stand Transfer

Rising from a low surface or getting out of a car can be difficult for a care-receiver. Care-receivers may make multiple attempts to stand up and often may fall backward into the car seat, chair, or bed. As with bed mobility, by applying good mechanics and leverage, this task can be made easier.

Caregivers typically do too much of the work in the sit-to-stand transfer. Many of you pull or lift up the care-receiver to standing, which makes it hard for you to keep the normal lumbar curve (neutral spine)—and it is simply too much work. Instead, position the care-receiver so that he can help the most. Try the following sequence:

1. *Position the care-receiver to the front of the chair*. If the care-receiver cannot move to the front of the chair on his own, lean him to one side, which off-loads the opposite hip. Pull the off-loaded hip forward, and then perform the same movement on the opposite side until the care-receiver is scooted to the front of the chair.

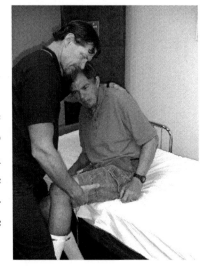

2. *Lean the care-receiver forward (nose past his toes).* The intent here is to get the care-receiver's center of gravity over his base of support—his feet—so that when he straightens out his legs, he will go straight up to standing. This is the part of the transfer where most caregivers perform too much of the work. Often, the care-receiver is not forward enough (his center of gravity is behind his base of support—his feet), so when he attempts to help with his legs, he actually drives his body back into the chair. The problem here is that the caregiver usually is in front, trying to pull up the care-receiver. This means that the caregiver is fighting against the care-receiver's push backwards and is trying to lift the care-receiver up at the same time, which not only is a lot of work but also puts strain on the caregiver's back. It is much easier to help the care-receiver forward and keep him forward as he attempts to push with his legs. With this strategy, the care-receiver does most of the work—which is good for all! The caregiver should stand on the

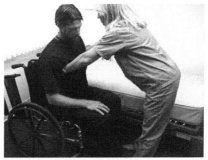

Incorrect: Pulling the care-receiver up to standing from the front

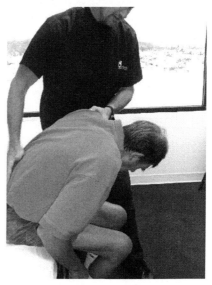

Correct: Assisting the care-receiver forward (nose past toes) with caregiver on side

side of the care-receiver, not in front of him, so that if the care-receiver needs a help up, the caregiver can give a little push from the side. (Being in front and trying to pull the care-receiver up is rough on the caregiver's back.) Remember, the lower the surface from which the care-receiver is getting up, the more forward he will need to go to get his center of gravity over his base of support.

Wheelchair-to-Bed Transfer

Standing pivot transfer. This transfer is used if the care-receiver is fairly strong and mobile (basically, someone who needs a little help with balance). As the caregiver, position yourself on the side opposite of the side to which he is transferring and gently guide the care-receiver over to the bed or chair.

Squat pivot transfer. This transfer is used if the care-receiver requires more assistance but can bear some weight through her legs. Position yourself in front of the care-receiver and assist the care-receiver forward (nose past toes) and close to your body. Hand placement can be up and over, or around and underneath the care-receiver's arms, depending on which position is most comfortable,

stable, and allows you to maintain the normal lumbar curve (neutral spine). The care-receiver's head and shoulder should be on the side *away* from the side to which he is being transferred. This is important, as by positioning the care-receiver this way, his hips are off-loaded on the side to which he is being transferred. This offers less resistance or friction. With this transfer, the care-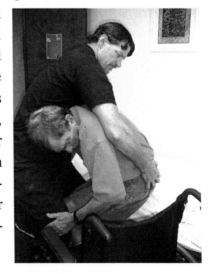

receiver always leads the transfer with the buttocks, not with the head and shoulders.

To complete this transfer, slowly rock the care-receiver forward and back, and on the count of three, rock forward, guiding the care-receiver's buttocks toward the chair or bed.

Dependent squat pivot transfer. This transfer is used when a care-receiver cannot bear weight or assist in the transfer at all. Examples of care-receivers for whom this transfer would be used are those affected by quadriplegia, paraplegia, and very dense hemiplegia. Dense hemiplegia refers to stroke survivors who have very little to no movement on the affected side of their bodies. The setup and positioning is the same as for the squat pivot transfer, described above. The care-receiver's legs will be in between the caregiver's knees, or the care-receiver's feet will be on the floor.

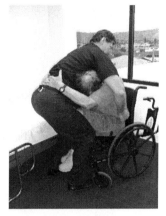

As the caregiver, you slowly rock forward and back with the care receiver tightly held against your body. On the count of three, rock the care-receiver forward while going back on your heels, and slide the care-receiver's buttocks toward the chair or bed.

By using leverage and good mechanics, your physical efforts will be minimized. It is important, however, that you are comfortable with your ability to safely perform this transfer. If you are of small stature, and the care-receiver is much larger (for example, 6'2" and weighing 220 pounds), then this may not be wise or safe. In that circumstance, you may need to consider other options, such as a mechanical lift, transfer board, or another person to assist.

Sliding board transfer. This is another type of dependent transfer for a care-receiver who cannot stand or bear any weight. It uses a sliding board, which basically creates a bridge between the two surfaces (from the wheelchair to the bed). Position the wheelchair close to the bed (or other surface to which the care-receiver is being transferred). If possible, remove the armrest on the side of the wheelchair that's facing the bed. Tilt the care-receiver to the opposite side, off-loading the hip so it is easier to slide the board securely under the hip. Once the board is in place, slowly rock forward and back, and on the count of three, rock the care-receiver forward while going back on your heels. Keep the care-receiver tightly against your body and slide the care-receiver's buttocks toward the bed.

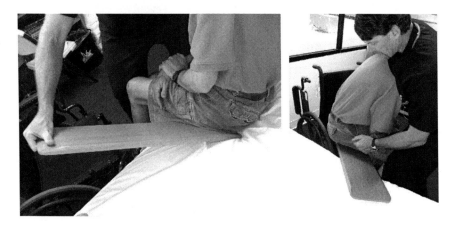

Two-person transfer. If it is too difficult or unsafe to transfer a care-receiver without assistance, another option is a two-person transfer. Other than obviously needing two people, the transfer is almost identical to the squat pivot transfer presented above. The first caregiver positions himself in front of the care-receiver (as shown on page 33). The second caregiver positions himself either behind the care-receiver or on the side to which the care-receiver is being transferred; he assists by placing his hands on the care-receiver's hips.

The first caregiver (usually the primary caregiver) counts to three, and the two caregivers work together. This transfer can be used with a sliding board as well.

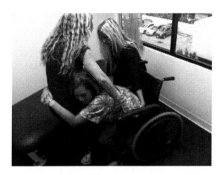

Mechanical lift transfer. This is a dependent transfer that allows one caregiver to perform a transfer with the use of a mechanical lift. A mechanical lift is an option to consider if you cannot protect your back or safely perform a manual transfer. The many different types of lifts on the market range from manual to hydraulic to electric. These different products vary greatly, and the "right" device depends on multiple factors, including whether the care-receiver needs something portable or fixed, and the cost of the device relative to the care-receiver's budget.

Although each type of mechanical device is slightly different from the others, they have some points in common. All devices have a sling to secure the care-receiver. The sling is usually secured to the care-receiver while she is in bed, and it typically stays underneath the care-receiver while she is in the wheelchair. To place the sling, have the care-receiver positioned on her side. Roll up half the sling and squish it as far as you can underneath the care-receiver. (This is similar to the way the draw sheet is placed.) Roll the care-receiver to the opposite side, and pull the sling through until it is completely under the care-receiver. The next step is to simply hook the sling to the mechanical lift, and you—and the care-receiver—are on your way. When lowering the care-receiver to a wheelchair, it is helpful to push him back in the chair as you are lowering him to minimize the need to pull him up, once he is positioned in the chair.

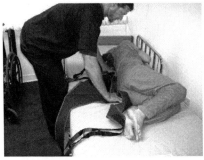
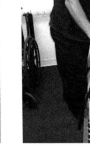

Mechanical lift: Positioning sling   Mechanical lift: Positioning sling

Repositioning in the wheelchair. Here is a familiar scene: The care-receiver is placed upright and in the middle of the chair. Thirty minutes later, he has scooted out of the chair toward the floor. Repositioning the care-receiver is, in many cases, a recurring necessity.

When pulling a care-receiver up in a chair from behind, do not take hold under the care-receiver's armpits. The shoulder joint is very mobile but not stable, so pulling up on this joint can cause injury. Also, a large bundle of nerves and blood vessels is located in the axilla (armpit), and pressure on them is uncomfortable and could cause injury. To pull a care-receiver up in a chair, it is best to take hold of the care-receiver's wrists while standing behind him. The care-receiver should now use his arms to press or squeeze your arms. This puts the most pressure on the care-receiver's flank (the sides of the upper trunk), which can tolerate more pressure and is less fragile than the skin on the forearms. You should be in a slightly squatting position, while keeping an arch in your low back. The final step is for you to straighten out your legs, pulling the care-receiver's buttocks to the back of the wheelchair seat.

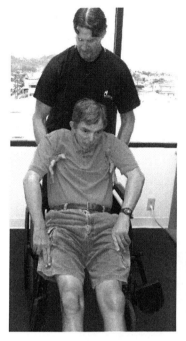 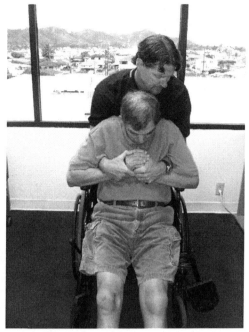

Incorrect wheelchair repositioning   Correct wheelchair repositioning

Floor Transfer

This is most likely the hardest of all transfers. If the care-receiver has fallen and is on the floor, first make sure that he did not sustain an injury. If you are uncertain whether he has been injured, or if you feel that he may be at risk for injury, it is best to call for help or call 911. In many cases, the care-receiver may simply slide out of bed or out of a chair, and it is clear that there is no injury. The sequence below illustrates a floor transfer in which the care-receiver can assist so you, the caregiver, do not have to lift dead weight and risk a back injury. If the care-receiver is unable to bear weight through his knees or you feel uncomfortable in your ability to safely perform this transfer, call for assistance.

1. Roll the care-receiver to his side, curled up into "fetal position."

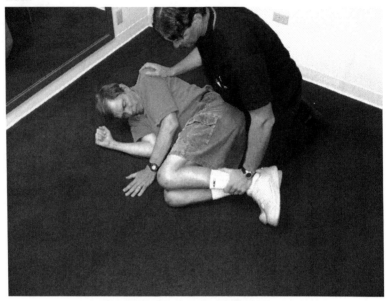

Floor transfer: Fetal position

2. Pull up on the care-receiver's top shoulder so that he can position his bottom arm to rest on his elbow.

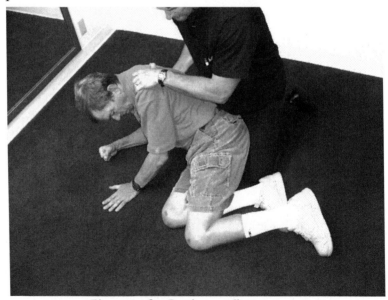

Floor transfer: Resting on elbow

3. Place your hands on the care-receiver's hips to assist in rolling him into the all-fours position (on his hands and knees).

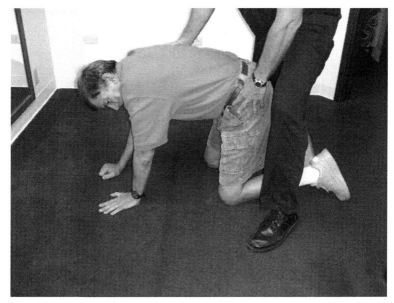

Floor transfer: All fours

4. From behind, gently pull the care-receiver's shoulders back and assist him so that he can "walk" his hands up his thigh until he is in "tall kneeling" position. If a chair, couch, or bed is close by, you can assist him in crawling or walking on all fours until he reaches the chair; then he can use his arms to assist himself to a tall kneeling position.

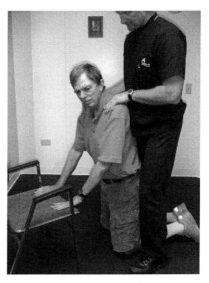

Floor transfer: Tall kneeling

5. From behind, assist the care-receiver in shifting his weight to one side, while the care-receiver positions his opposite knee forward to get into the "half-kneeling" position.

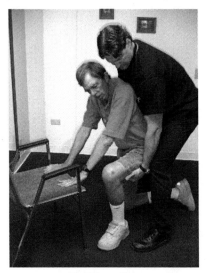

Half-kneeling

6. Now assist the care-receiver in leaning forward from the hip, over the front leg, so that his weight is over the front leg.

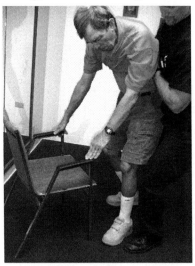

Floor transfer: Half-kneel to stand

7. Finally, gently pull the care-receiver up, while he is pushing up with his leg, until both legs are firmly beneath him, and he is standing tall.

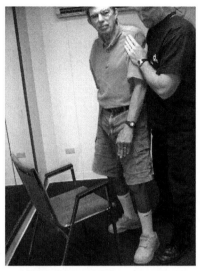

Completion of floor transfer

Car Transfer

One of the toughest transfers can be getting a care-receiver in and out of a vehicle. Manual wheelchair transfers to a vehicle can involve a lot of hard work because there is so little space in which to operate. The principles for car transfers are the same as the other transfers mentioned. Remember to always keep your normal lumbar curve to protect your back, despite any circumstances. Helpful hints and strategies to make car transfers easier and safer are presented below.

If the care-receiver has difficulty bearing weight through his legs, a sliding board transfer works well for a car transfer. A sliding board serves as a bridge from the wheelchair to the car, but its effectiveness depends on the make of the vehicle—a sliding board works fine when the car's seat is on about the same level as the wheelchair, but it doesn't work well for SUVs or other taller vehicles. The sequence for this type of transfer is as follows:

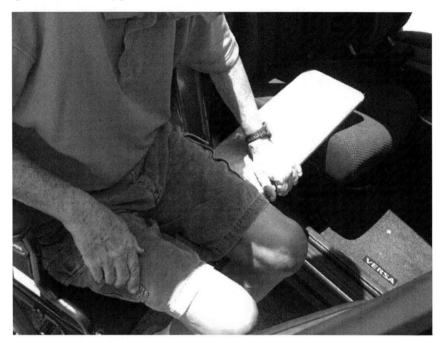

Wheelchair to car sliding board transfer

Step # 1—Vehicle position. The primary concern is the level of the transfer surfaces. It is quite challenging to transfer "uphill" on a sliding board to get into a van, truck, or SUV. Not much can be done to a vehicle to change the ground-to-seat height, other than getting a different car, which is not practical. If you, as the caregiver, are in need of a replacement vehicle, however, the ground-to-seat height should be one consideration. Other considerations are four doors versus two doors, but the style of car door that allows for the most room and the most level transfer heights is best.

One strategy for transferring from a wheelchair to a higher vehicle seat is to park next to a curb so that the wheelchair is a curb's height closer to the vehicle seat. Most curbs average four inches in height, so this strategy would decrease the ascent upward to the vehicle seat by four inches. The reverse setup may be best when the transfer is from out of the vehicle to the wheelchair. In this circumstance, positioning the vehicle on the opposite side of the curb can take advantage of gravity so that the care-receiver can slide downhill, which should be an easier transfer.

Step # 2—Preparing your vehicle. Another consideration is whether the transfer should be into the front seat or backseat. The seat that allows you the most room and best advantage is the one you should use. This will vary greatly, based on make and model of the vehicle. Some vehicles have built-in handles above the door in the front seat, but some back seats allow for a wider door opening and therefore better, closer positioning of the wheelchair. Whichever is easiest is the right choice. Regardless of which seat, front or back, you need to prepare the vehicle as much as possible. If transferring into the front seat, it is usually advantageous to push the seat as far back as possible to allow more leg room. The reverse is true when transferring to the backseat—push the front seat up as far forward as possible. Also, if the care-receiver has difficulty with bending her legs to get into the vehicle, recline the seat back, if possible, to allow for more room for the legs to swing in or out. If the care-receiver has total hip precautions (can't bend the hip past 90 degrees; can't cross midline; can't point toes inward), then it's necessary to recline the seat to avoid bending past 90 degrees.

Step # 3—Positioning of the caregiver/transfer preparation. On a manual chair, remove all of the movable parts on the side that is being transferred. This includes the footrest and armrest—the fewer obstacles, the better. Wedging yourself between the door and the car is not the best approach—it allows you very little room and will ultimately put you in a position where you will lose your normal lumbar curve. There are better strategies so that you can be close enough to give the assistance needed without getting stuck in the process of the transfer. One option is to park the wheelchair against the car door into which you are transferring. From behind the chair, you will be on the left side, between the chair and the car. This allows for the wheelchair to be wedged against the door and provides a stable surface for the care-receiver to hold on to.

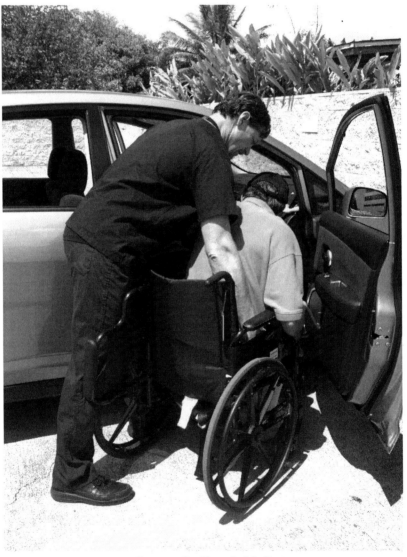

Car transfer (from behind)

Another option is for you to be wedged between the open door and the wheelchair but not in front of the chair. In this way, you can control the stability of the door (i.e., making sure it won't move or close while transferring into the car). This option will only work if the make and model of the car and the size of the parking space allows for enough room when the door is fully opened to accommodate you, the chair, and the care-receiver.

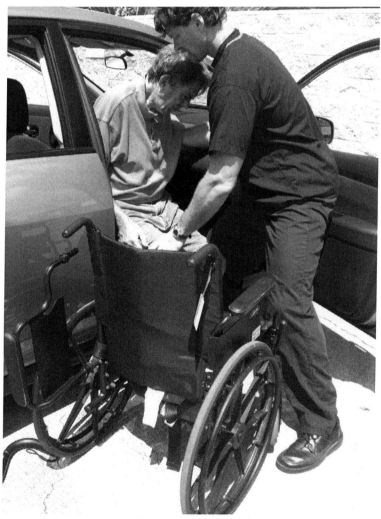

Car transfer (in front)

A third option is for you to assist from inside the car. You would assist the care-receiver to standing; he would then hold on to the door while you come around and enter the car on the driver's side to assist with directing the care-receiver's buttocks to the car seat.

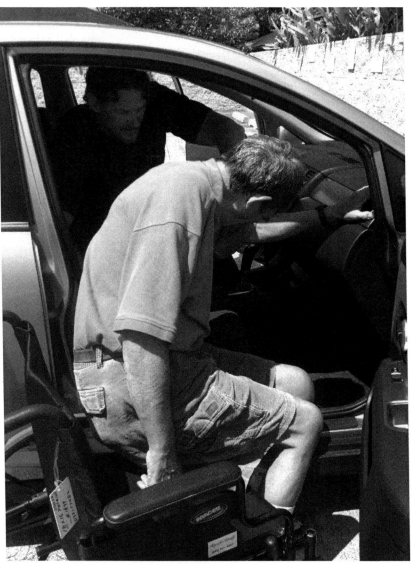

Car transfer (from in car)

Step # 4—Scooting/positioning in car seat. The steering wheel is a sturdy "grab-bar" to help scoot. The hand-hold that some cars have above the door can assist as well. If the care-receiver can pull or push herself up, the caregiver (from the driver's side) can help scoot the buttocks into the center of the seat by taking hold of the hips or transfer belt. You also could have a towel on the car seat prior to the transfer so that you can use it to pull the buttocks more squarely in the seat.

Transferring or Lifting a Manual Wheelchair into the Car

Step # 1
Push the wheelchair to the back of the car (trunk should be open) and lock the back wheels.

Step # 2
Grasp the front and the back portion of the seat and pull straight up. This move is quite simple, but it may need a gentle shake to get it going. As the sling seat is pulled up, the sides (rails) will come together, folding the chair.
Note: The best way to manage unfolding the wheelchair is to set the chair down on its wheels and push down on the two side rails.

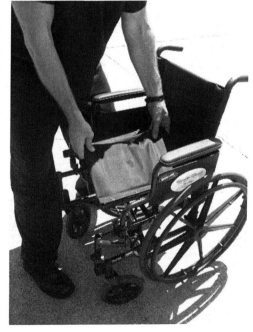

Step # 3

Place the chair parallel to the back bumper. While bending your knees and keeping your back straight, lean the top part of the locked wheels that are closest to you onto your mid-thigh, and grab the locked wheels at the 10:00 and 2:00 position. Using your legs as the pivot fulcrum, pull the chair upward, allowing it to pivot on your thigh to clear the front of the chair over the bumper and trunk threshold.

Using this leverage, you will be surprised how much more manageable the wheelchair becomes.

If it is still too difficult for you to place the wheelchair into the trunk, there are different mechanical lifts made to fit trunks for this particular transfer.

Navigating Thresholds and Other Obstacles to Wheelchairs

Thresholds. The threshold is the piece of wood or metal that lies under a door; it can vary in height. Thresholds can be difficult to roll over because they are typically raised higher than the floor. Wheelchairs with large front casters can climb thresholds more easily than those with small front casters. If thresholds are a problem when pushing the care-receiver in her wheelchair, try the following:

- Push the wheelchair forward until the front casters rest against the threshold.
- Tip the wheelchair back slightly, moving the casters up and over threshold.

Ramps. A standard ramp should have a grade no steeper than a 1:12 ratio. This means that for every inch of rise (increase in height), there should be 12 inches of grade or slope. Using this formula, a ramp leading to a door with two 8-inch steps would be 16 feet long.

Many ramps, however, are much steeper due to space constraints. When pushing the wheelchair up a ramp, make sure that the anti-tippers are down so that the wheelchair will not flip backward. When ascending a steep ramp, have the care-receiver lean forward as you push to minimize the tendency for the chair to tip backwards (this also makes it easier for you to push). When descending a ramp, have the care-receiver lean back to minimize the likelihood of his falling forward out of the chair. For really steep descents, a better option might be to guide the wheelchair down backwards; in this case, the care-receiver leans forward as you ease the wheelchair slowly down the ramp.

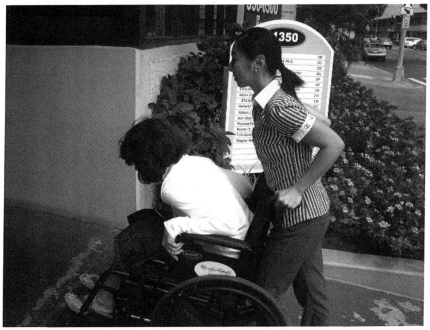

Ascending ramp

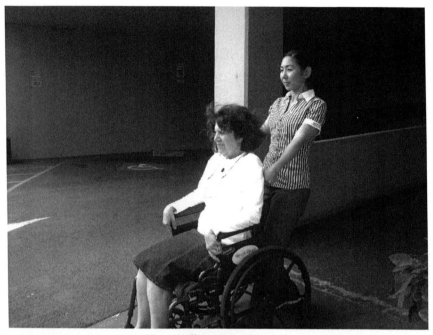

Descending ramp, forward

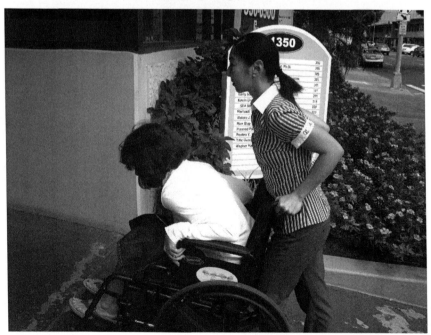

Descending ramp, backward

Curbs. If curb cuts are missing, in poor repair, or blocked, you may need to negotiate the care-receiver and wheelchair over a curb. To ascend a curb, follow this sequence:

- Push the front casters against the curb.
- Tilt the wheelchair/care-receiver backwards to lift the front casters onto the curb. Rest the back of the chair on your thighs if you don't have the arm strength.
- Once the casters are resting on the curb, the care-receiver should lean forward as you push the chair forward so that the back wheels roll over the curb and up onto the sidewalk.

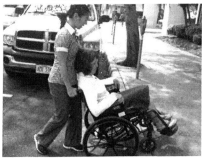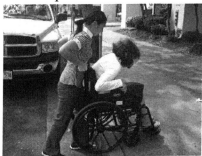

To descend a curb, follow this sequence:
- Turn the care-receiver and wheelchair so that it is backwards, back wheels facing the curb.
- Slowly roll the wheelchair backwards as the care-receiver leans forward, until the back wheels are in contact with the street.
- The care-receiver now should lean back as you slowly lower the front casters down to the street.

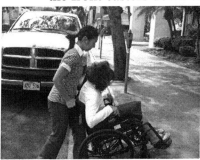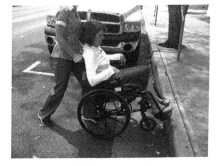

CHAPTER FIVE:

ADAPTIVE DEVICES FOR EASIER DAILY LIVING

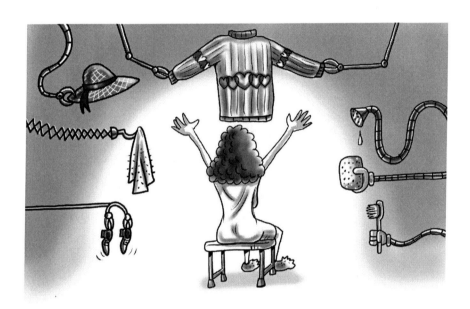

Activities of daily living are just that—daily—so it is appropriate to look at some common problems and adaptive devices and strategies that may be helpful for the care-receiver. The devices covered in this chapter are not all-inclusive—there are many more. See the appendix for resources and help in searching for assistive devices.

Grooming. An electric razor increases safety and ease of shaving. Larger handle hairbrushes and toothbrushes are easier to grip. If the care-receiver is having difficulty controlling fine movements, an electric toothbrush can help with thoroughly brushing teeth.

Upper-Extremity Dressing. If the care-receiver has a problem with posture or balance, he may find it easier to sit while putting on a shirt or sweater. If one arm is more rigid or has less range of motion than the other, it is usually easier to dress that side first. Loose-fitting clothing, larger buttons, and Velcro fasteners are some helpful options. If the care-receiver has difficulty removing a blouse or shirt, it may be easier to undress by grabbing the shirt from behind the neck and pulling it over the head. Buttoning is often difficult for care-receivers, and many people find that a button aid is helpful. A button aid allows a care-receiver who does not have good fine-motor control to button a shirt or blouse. The wide-grip handle has a wire extension that hooks on a button and allows the button to be pulled through the buttonhole.

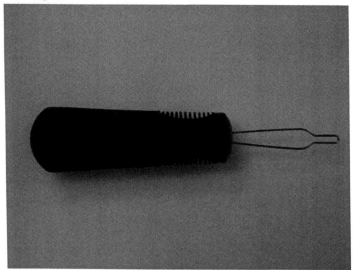

Button aid

Lower-Extremity Dressing. It is usually safer and easier for the care-receiver to put her feet into shorts or pants while leaning against a wall or while sitting. If the care-receiver has difficulty reaching down to the feet, a "reacher," or dressing stick, can help to get the pant legs over the feet. A reacher is a device that has a grasp-handle on one end and a grabber on the other that allows a care-receiver to reach and grab objects that are lower or higher than his arm's reach. A dressing stick also allows for an extended reach but uses a hook at one end versus the dynamic grabber that the reacher has. Various styles of sock aids may help to get the feet into the socks. To use a sock aid, the care-receiver pulls the sock over an open trough and then places his foot down and in the sock as he pulls the sock aid up and out of the sock. A long-handled shoehorn is helpful for putting on shoes. Velcro closures make fastening shoes easier; and elastic shoelaces can convert a laced-shoe into a slip-on shoe.

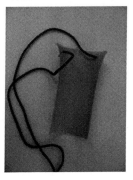

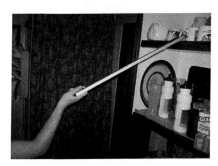

Reacher

Dressing stick

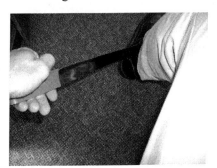

Sock aid

Long-handled shoehorn

Bathing. Grab-bars in the tub or shower can help with entering and exiting safely. It is best to have the grab-bars installed by a contractor or by someone knowledgeable in construction. A rubber mat or non-skid decals on the tub or shower floor can help to prevent slips and falls. Sitting on a bath bench to bathe also helps if the care-receiver has problems with balance or has difficulty reaching his feet. "Soap on a rope" keeps soap within reach and prevents the care-receiver from dropping it. Liquid soap and shampoo in pump bottles may also be easier to manage. Bath brushes and sponges can help to reach the back and feet when washing.

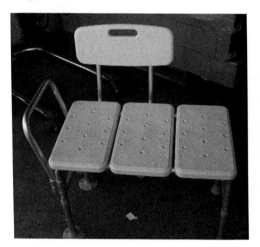 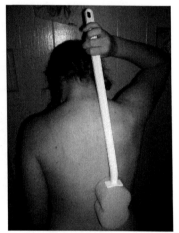

Bath bench   Long-handled sponge

Eating. Tremors and weakness can interfere with eating. Some people find that weighted utensils help to control the tremors. Also, angled utensils make scooping and inserting food into the mouth easier and neater. In addition, a plate guard creates a ledge on a plate against which food can be scooped, and it prevents spillage. If the care-receiver has difficulty cutting up food, a rocker knife may be used. The rocker knife has a rounded sharp end (rocker) with a wide-grip handle on top that allows the care-receiver to cut with one hand, rather than using a knife and fork and cutting by performing a sawing motion, which takes two hands.

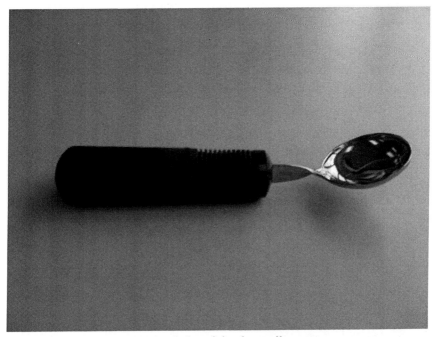

Angled, weighted utensil

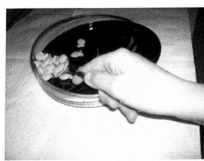
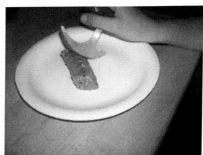

Plate guard   Rocker knife

Meal Preparation. It is helpful to organize the kitchen so that frequently used items are placed within reach (as close to waist-height as possible). A "reacher" can be used to pick up objects from the floor or from a high shelf. A rubberized shelf liner or a wet dishcloth placed under bowls, pans, and cutting boards will stabilize them during food preparation.

Some cutting boards have raised edges to keep food from falling off the board, and some have small nails on the surface, which help to stabilize food while slicing or chopping. An electric can opener is an easy solution if the care-receiver has difficulty opening cans. Different types of jar openers can be useful as well, such as the rounded rubber disc that allows for a better grasp, or a jar opener with a handle that requires less grip strength to use.

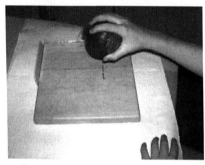

Spiked cutting board

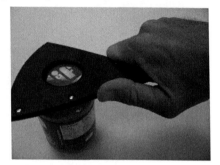

Jar opener

CHAPTER SIX:

ASSISTIVE DEVICES

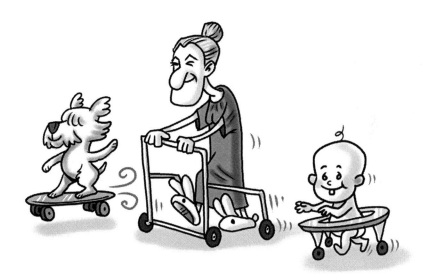

Ideally, recommendations for assistive devices should come from a physical therapist or physician. The needs of the care-receiver, however, may change, so that the original recommendations may no longer be completely appropriate. Sometimes, an appropriate device is recommended but the care-receiver does not use it correctly.

In most circumstances, assistive devices are covered by Medicare and other insurers with a physician's order. In order to bill the insurance for these items, it is best to work with a durable medical equipment (DME) supplier, rather than purchasing the item with cash at a drugstore. Local physical therapists or physicians should be a good resource for reputable DME suppliers in the area.

A spectrum of assisted devices is available, from minimal support to greater support. The timing of when and which device the care-receiver may require depends on his specific needs. For orthopedic issues, most care-receivers use assistive devices to decrease weight-bearing through a particular leg. This could be due to pain or weakness from osteoarthritis in a hip or knee; a post-surgical condition, such as hip, knee, or ankle injury; or the inability to weight-bear on one side of the body following a stroke. With conditions such as Parkinson's disease, it often is an issue of balance, rather than the need to bear less weight through the legs. The following section presents the profiles of two specific devices.

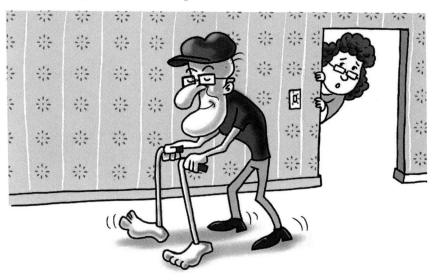

Canes. A single-point cane is helpful for multiple reasons. It can provide minimal support for balance and can assist in walking. When used by care-receivers with hemiparesis or orthopedic injuries, the cane is used on the opposite side of the injured leg. Many times, people with Parkinson's disease use the cane with the involved arm to promote arm swing and to re-engage that affected arm into the walking pattern. A single-point cane also can be helpful with transitions through thresholds and elevators by blocking the door. Other types of canes can give more support if the care-receiver needs to weight-bear more through the arms and less through one of the legs. These types of canes include a small-base quad cane, large-base quad cane, and hemi-walker. These devices can work well for orthopedic cases and hemiparesis, but they may not be useful at all for people with Parkinson's disease, as these canes are too clumsy and difficult to manage for those with a movement disorder.

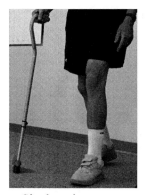
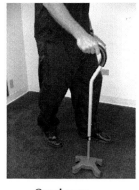
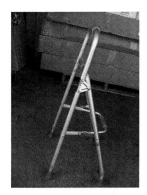

Single-point cane   Quad cane   Hemi-walker

Walkers. Walkers are useful if the support needed is greater than that offered by a cane; however, walkers can promote bad posture and an unnatural walking pattern. With a walker, there is a tendency for the care-receiver to stoop or indulge in "forward posturing," which places the center of gravity (the shoulders and head) in front of the base of support (the feet)—the walker almost forces this posture. The walker also completely takes away arm swing. Arm swing plays a major role in assuring an efficient walking pattern by promoting pelvic rotation. Without pelvic rotation, there is a more lateral quality to the gait, much like the image of Frankenstein's monster, which is harder on the joints and not as efficient. Pick-up–style walkers are rarely recommended. The pick-up–style walker has four tips so the care-receiver must pick up the walker to advance it. This requires the care-receiver to be able to stand on his own two legs without support while the walker is moving. The most common recommendation is the front-wheeled rolling walker. This walker is easier to maneuver because it does not have to be picked up to advance it forward. Even with a walker, the care-receiver should try to walk with a step-through gait rather than a step-to gait. He should step *past* the opposite foot (a step-through gait), rather than stepping even with the foot (a step-to gait). The step-through gait pattern is the normal walking pattern. It is also important for the care-receiver to try to step into the walker, which means that he shouldn't bend over too much, with the walker too far in front of him. If the care-receiver steps into the walker with each step, he will keep a better posture. Another style of walker is the four-wheeled walker, which typically comes with hand brakes and a fold-down seat. A four-wheeled walker can move too much as it has four swivel-style wheels that can roll in any direction; at times, it may have a tendency to get away from the user. The care-receiver should try using this type of walker before purchase.

The height of the walker should also be considered. Most physical therapists will set the height of a walker (and a cane) by having the care-receiver stand tall, with arms relaxed down his sides. The walker is then raised or lowered until the handle is at or close to the bend of the wrist. The height can be adjusted for comfort by moving the extension tubes up or down one hole. This strategy allows for the most optimal leverage for the arms to weight-bear. The traditional use of walkers for orthopedic injuries is for weight-bearing through the arms, so the arms do more work and lessen the burden of the injured leg. This situation typically is not the case with care-receivers who are affected by Parkinson's disease (PD). For these care-receivers, it is better to raise the walker much higher than the bend of the wrist—this will aid in posture. Care-receivers with PD most likely will use the walker for balance more than for decreasing weight-bearing through the legs.

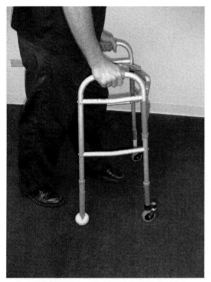

Front-wheeled rolling walker

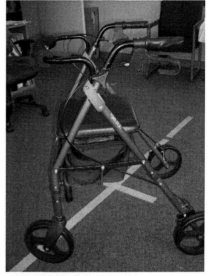

Four-wheeled walker

One alternative to assistive devices that is worth mentioning is a hiking pole or walking stick. This device has caught on recently as a fitness option for seniors. It offers support for balance but also aids in a normal walking pattern because it mimics arm swing. I use these devices frequently when working with clients who have Parkinson's disease (see www.parkinsonsmoveit.com). Some care-receivers may like this alternative as it does not look like a medical device. Walking poles are available at most sporting goods stores.

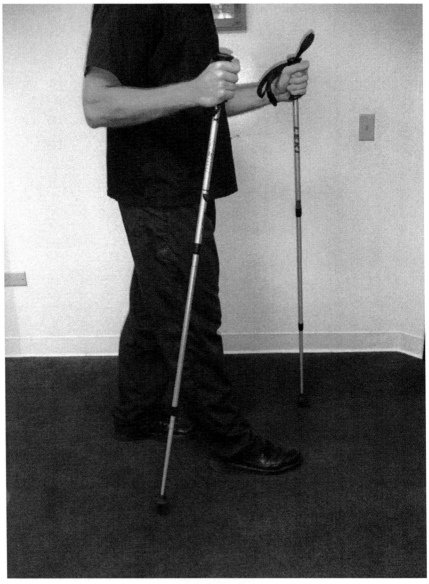

Walking poles

CHAPTER SEVEN:

FALL PREVENTION AND FALL-PROOFING THE HOME

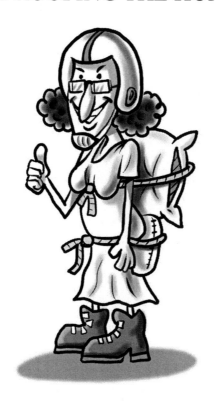

Falls and the consequences of falls, such as hip fractures, can be devastating to care-receivers and their families. Often, the consequences of falls prevent care-receivers from living independently at home. Injury from falls is the sixth leading cause of death in people over sixty-five years of age, causing more deaths than pneumonia or diabetes each year in this age group. In the United States, approximately 10,000 deaths each year are related to falls, and the majority of these are related to hip fractures. Despite the statistics, falls often can be prevented by "fall-proofing" the care-receiver's home and by changing or compensating for factors that lead to falls.

The following risk factors are associated with falls in the home:

- People older than seventy-five years of age: Care-receivers older than seventy-five typically show more physical decline, such as decreased strength, and complicating health factors, such as osteoarthritis and vision decline that places them at greater risk for falls.
- Use of an assistive device: Care-receivers who rely on the use of canes and walkers are shown to have higher risk for falls due to some type of physical decline.
- Chronic neuromuscular conditions, such as Parkinson's disease, stroke, etc.: These conditions show different levels of physical decline, which place care-receivers at greater risk for falls than people of same age group without a chronic condition.
- Use of medications (especially the use of four or more prescription drugs)
- Previous fall history
- Reduced vision: Vision is one of the three primary balance factors. A decline in vision places the care-receiver at greater fall risk because he will rely on one less balance factor.
- Environmental hazards: This includes anything in the environment that can create a hazard or barrier, such as throw-rugs that can cause tripping, stairs, etc.
- Deconditioned state/generalized weakness: A decline in strength places a care-receiver at greater risk for falls. This commonly is seen following a hospitalization or recovery

from an ailment, such as the flu or a cold, which forces a care-receiver to be bed-bound, even for a few days.

- Postural hypotension: Postural hypotension is low blood pressure when going from lying or sitting to a standing position. Low blood pressure can cause light-headedness or, in severe cases, cause a care-receiver to pass out.

The common factors that affect balance and either prevent or lead to falls relate to the care-receiver's physical capabilities and characteristics (intrinsic factors) and those that relate to the care-receiver's environment (extrinsic factors).

Intrinsic Factors
The three primary **intrinsic factors** are vision, sensation (somatosensory), and vestibular system.

Vision. Age-related changes in vision can decrease the ability to accurately perceive changes in surface conditions or the presence of hazards in the environment. Eye conditions such as cataracts, glaucoma, and macular degeneration among older adults have been associated with an increasing rate of falls. Regular eye exams can decrease risk of falls for care-receivers by minimizing visual deficits, allowing for better anticipation of the changes in surfaces and helping to perceive environmental hazards, such as negotiating curbs, stairs, and uneven terrain.

Sensation. The somatosensory system provides information about the spatial relationship of the body to the support surface. It refers to the ability to feel the surface, whether it's the firm surface of wood floors or the soft surface of a padded carpet. In the absence of or decline in vision, the ability to feel the surface becomes the primary source of sensory information to aid in balance and in moving around in dark areas (for example, trying to negotiate down a dark hallway to the bathroom in the middle of the night). Sensation is the care-receiver's primary asset in preventing falls. There are times when sensation is disrupted, such as when walking on uneven ground. When this occurs, the care-receiver has to rely more on the other two factors to avoid falling.

Vestibular system. This is the balance system that is housed in the inner ear and is activated when the care-receiver moves his head. The vestibular system becomes very important when the other two systems are impaired. Examples are when one is walking on uneven terrain, which disrupts the somatosensory system, or the ability to feel, in conjunction with being in really crowded or darker areas that can distort vision. The vestibular system can be trained to better compensate for visual and/or sensory deficits with specific exercises that a physical therapist can teach. Balance exercises can improve the vestibular system, which forces it to adapt and become stronger and more responsive.

Other Intrinsic Factor

Posture/osteoporosis: Good posture is critical to good balance; posture refers to the body's alignment. With age, some people develop a hump in the upper back, known as a "kyphotic posture." This postural change moves the center of gravity of the body, making the care-receiver more susceptible to falling backwards when walking up a ramp or reaching overhead, or for falling forward when walking down a ramp.

Even though care-receivers may not have control over certain intrinsic factors, such as macular degeneration, risks of falling can be greatly decreased if the care-receiver recognizes his physical limitations and at-risk situations, as well as training his body to compensate for impairments in one or more of the balance systems.

Extrinsic Factors

Extrinsic factors also can affect the care-receiver's risk of falls. The two primary external risk factors are medications and the physical environment.

Medications. If the care-receiver is taking four or more prescription medications, he is at higher risk for falls. Certain medications have side effects that can contribute to fall risk, as can the interactions of some drugs and supplements, which can cause adverse effects. Certain classes of prescription medication are associated with higher fall risk than others. These include sedatives/hypnotics, antidepressants, and psychotropic medications. It is highly recommended that you, as the caregiver, keep a consolidated drug list for the primary care physician or any specialist so that he is aware of the medications that the care-receiver is taking and does not prescribe a medication that may cause an adverse reaction. It is common for care-receivers to have several specialists—orthopedist, neurologist, rheumatologists, urologist, etc.—who may prescribe a medication for an ailment under their specialty. Unless the care-receiver is part of a closed health-care system that has all of this information available as a common file, communication from one specialist to another does not typically happen. The various specialists may not be aware of all of the medications that the care-receiver is taking. It is best to keep an updated medication list or put all of the supplements and prescription medications in a bag and take it to the primary care physician or pharmacist to review. The primary care physician and pharmacist are more likely to take a global view of all of the medications and may be in a better position to pick up on any interactions that may cause trouble. It is a matter of looking at the forest instead of a tree. Most pharmacies offer free medication review.

Environment. The second external factor that can have direct impact on fall risk is the physical environment itself. Homes have many hazards, including floor rugs that are not secured down, exposed electrical or appliance cords, poor lighting, lack of grab-bars in the bathroom, general clutter, too-soft plush carpeting, absence of night-lights, cabinets that are too high, furniture that is too low, and raised thresholds into different rooms.

The following list offers simple home-safety strategies (see chapter eight for more comprehensive information):

- Lighting. Make sure corridors are well lighted.
- Night-lights. Use of night-lights can aid vision in the middle of the night.
- Throw rugs. Get rid of throw rugs, or secure them down with two-way carpet tape.
- Clutter. Reduce clutter at least to have clear walking paths.
- Toilets. Use a raised toilet seat and/or install grab-bars next to the toilet. Tall commodes are available as well and are more stable than a raised toilet seat.
- Place a bathmat outside the shower. Safety grid or rubber-brush mats provide secure traction on wet surfaces, are stiffer than a throw rug.
- Many bathtubs have sliding glass doors. Remove these and replace them with a shower curtain rod and shower curtain.
- When balance and strength are an issue, a tub transfer bench eliminates stepping in and out and allows easy access to the tub from the seated position at all times. This will not work with a glass-door shower or in a shower-only stall. A shower or tub chair also is an option; it fits entirely inside the tub or shower, but the care-receiver must be able to step into the tub.
- Smart placement of the grab-bar is essential. Avoid diagonal grab-bar placement, as this can allow frail hands to slip downward. Place the bar horizontally when it's needed for pulling up from a seated position. Place the bar vertically for

assistance with stepping in and out of the tub.

- Cabinets. Store items in lower areas or redesign cabinets to be lower or accessible without the need of a step stool.

- Low seats. Make sure there is at least one chair that has a higher seat-to-floor height from which the care-receiver can rise without difficulty. Lift chairs are also available on the market. These chairs are spring-loaded and assist a care-receiver to standing.

- Heavily padded plush carpet. This type of carpet disrupts *proprioception*—the care-receiver's ability to feel where she is walking, which places her at greater risk for falls. Replace padded plush carpets with low-pile carpet, tile, or wooden flooring.

Another Fall-Prevention Strategy: Exercise!

Regular physical exercise can greatly reduce risk for falls. Studies show that older adults who exhibit greater quadriceps strength have a reduced risk for falls compared to older adults with lesser muscle strength in the same muscle groups. General physical condition can affect risk for falls. It is very common for care-receivers to experience loss of balance and/or falls following prolonged bed rest or hospitalization. In these circumstances, the muscles experience weakness and may atrophy, and the vestibular system is not as efficient when it is not challenged or stressed due to inactivity.

In addition to monitoring the care-receiver's medications and physical environment to ensure proper balance, encouraging exercise and activity can help to restore or improve balance. Three different exercise routines are included in this book to assist in decreasing risk for falls. (See chapters eleven, twelve, and thirteen.)

CHAPTER EIGHT:

AFFORDABLE HOME ADAPTATIONS

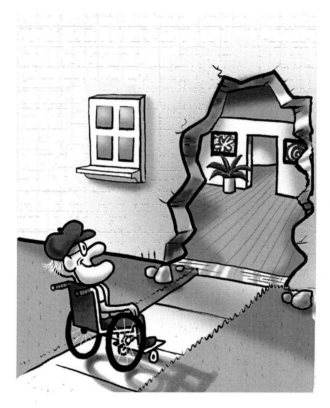

Caregivers often adapt to the care-receiver's physical environment by trying to work around obstacles. This chapter will present ways to make the home more accessible. Many changes can be made to the home—without expensive renovations—that can alleviate frustration (for example, installing a handheld shower head). Some of the changes will seem small but can be essential to greater independence for the care-receiver and will provide less physical stress on you as the caregiver.

Getting into Your Home

- If the care-receiver is a wheelchair user, consider installing a curb-cut so that you can more easily maneuver the wheelchair without as much lifting, which may put a strain on your back.
- A parking space with an adjacent four-foot aisle allows for a wheelchair to maneuver alongside the car.
- If there are stairs at the entry, ramps with a non-skid surface can make getting into the home much easier. Prefabricated ramps may work, depending on the slope and available space; otherwise, consider a custom-built ramp.
- If the care-receiver is ambulatory, a good handrail to assist in negotiating the stairs may be all he needs. A good handrail is one that the care-receiver can wrap his hands around.
- Is the front door wide enough to accommodate a wheelchair? A door with at least a 32-inch opening allows a wheelchair or walker to pass through it. An inexpensive "swing-clear hinge" can widen a doorway up to 1½ inches.
- Can the care-receiver manage the door handle? If the care-receiver (or caregiver) struggles with arthritic hands or has any difficulty with the hands, a lever or loop-type of handle can be installed in place of a round knob that requires twisting and much hand strength.
- Consider a beveled or flat threshold at the entry, which won't trip a foot or block a wheelchair.
- If space allows, a bench should be placed outside the door to hold packages while opening the door.

Kitchen

Safety

- A stove design with the control knobs on the front is safer than the traditional style with the knobs in the back. A front design allows both the care-receiver and you to more easily reach the controls and to avoid crossing an arm over hot burners.
- Install a lever-handle faucet in the sink, with built-in anti-scald protection.
- Only use step stools that have a non-slip surface.

Simplify

- Knob handles for drawers and cabinets can be replaced by C-shaped or D-shaped handles, which take less hand dexterity to manipulate.
- A lazy Susan can be used in a cabinet to bring items around to the front; or install pull-out shelving.
- An open drawer can provide a low work surface when a cutting board is placed over it. An open drawer also can be used to hold a bowl.
- A rolling cart is useful for storing items within easy reach for the care-receiver, and it offers leg space under it so that the care-receiver can sit next to it to perform meal preparations. Removing a shelf door allows for leg room under a counter.
- Use the highest wattage bulb approved for the fixtures to increase the lighting around the stove, sink, and work areas.

Bathroom

Safety

- Care-receivers often need to use the bathroom at night, but limited vision in the dark will place the care-receiver at greater risk for falls. A simple solution is use a night-light.

- Place non-slip strips or decals in the bathtub and on the shower floor for better traction.
- Grab-bars by the bathroom sink and toilet will assist in safe transfers. Do not rely on towel racks as grab-bars, as they are not designed for weight-bearing and will likely break or pull out of the wall if used in this manner.
- Lever-handle faucets with built-in anti-scald protection are also appropriate for the bathroom sink and the tub.
- Insulate hot water pipes underneath the sink, if they are exposed.
- Set the water heater to 120 degrees to avoid scalding.
- Unplug all electrical appliances (such as a hairdryer or electric razor) when not in use, and never use any electrical appliance near a filled sink or tub.

Simplify
- A raised toilet seat can make sitting and standing much easier, or install a tall commode.
- A handheld shower head allows the care-receiver to shower while sitting or standing.
- Use bath chairs or bath benches if balance in standing is a problem.
- Single-lever faucets are helpful for many care-receivers, as they require less hand dexterity.

Bedroom
- Closet poles and shelves should be at a height that can be easily reached, especially for wheelchair users.
- Firmer mattresses tend to be better for the back and usually make it easier for the care-receiver to move in bed.
- Rearrange furniture to allow for clear, wide passageways.

Living Areas

- Rearrange furniture to allow for clear, wide passageways.
- Place all cords along the wall, where they cannot cause tripping.
- Remove throw rugs or use double-sided carpet tape to secure rugs.
- Install a telephone jack close to a favorite chair and the bed to improve accessibility, or use a cordless phone.
- Make sure that the height of the care-receiver's chairs are high enough to allow for easy sit-to-standing. Chairs with arms can help with sit-to-standing as well. Care-receivers should avoid low, soft couches, as it's difficult to rise from them.

Laundry Room

- A front-opening washer/dryer is easier for the care-receiver to use than a traditional top-loading style.
- Having a table for folding clothes near the dryer reduces the number of times the care-receiver will have to move his laundry.

Larger-Scale Modifications

Sometimes larger-scale modifications are needed for the care-receiver to safely reside in the home, especially if he or she has a change in or decline in mobility (for example, needing a wheelchair after being ambulatory). While larger-scale modifications, such as widening doorways or other structural changes, are more costly and require hiring a contractor, they can make a home dramatically more livable and accessible. Adaptive construction requires attention to the personal needs of both the care-receiver and caregiver, rather than adherence to standard solutions. A contractor's license is not necessary for some smaller projects, such as installing grab-bars, but for larger projects, it's important to hire someone with a contractor's license. Below are some considerations for hiring a licensed contractor who will best address your needs:

- Some contractors have experience in home adaptation or in "barrier-free" construction for a commercial space, which may provide useful insight.
- Get referrals from trusted people or organizations.
- The local Better Business Bureau and Consumer Protection Office can provide information on whether anyone has filed a complaint against a particular contractor, and if so, how it was resolved.
- Get estimates in writing from several contractors. The estimates should detail the materials to be used, labor charges, the start and end dates, and total cost of the project.
- Don't pay the final bill until the work is completed.

See the Home Assessment Checklist in the Appendix for a checklist of all areas of the home with potential problems. This checklist offers solutions to each problem, which range from small adaptations to larger-scale modifications.

CHAPTER NINE:

WHEELCHAIRS

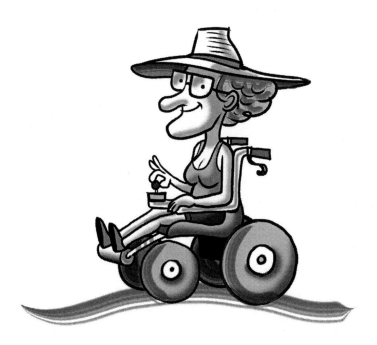

Types of Wheelchairs

If wheelchair mobility is the primary or only means of locomotion for the care-receiver, several needs should be considered when prescribing mobility devices and seating systems. It's not as simple as sending a friend or relative out to the drugstore to bring home a wheelchair. To maximize independence for the care-receiver and to minimize secondary health risk, such as skin breakdown or orthopedic injuries, the wheelchair needs to fit the care-receiver specifically, rather than the care-receiver's fitting the wheelchair. Ideally, a professional, such as a physical or occupational therapist, should assess the overall needs. A letter of justification from the care-receiver's physician, occupational therapist, or physical therapist often is required for reimbursement or coverage from insurers such as Medicare.

The more knowledge you have going into this process, the more you, as a caregiver, can guide and direct the process to assure that the needs of the care-receiver are met.

Some considerations when selecting a wheelchair include the following:

- Type of transfers
- Transportability—folding vs. rigid, power vs. manual
- Terrain
- Architectural barriers
- Cost and what is reimbursed by insurance

Manual wheelchairs can vary greatly in cost. At the time of this publication, most range between $200 and $4,000, depending on the model and features. Manual wheelchairs are offered in the following basic models:

Folding frame wheelchair

This conventional wheelchair is constructed with an X-shaped brace at the center that allows the frame to fold sideways. Folding an X-frame is simple, but the folding frame wheelchair is often heavy, and some caregivers are unable to load it into a vehicle without help. A standard-sized folding wheelchair averages between 28 and 32 pounds (sometimes more).

Transport wheelchair

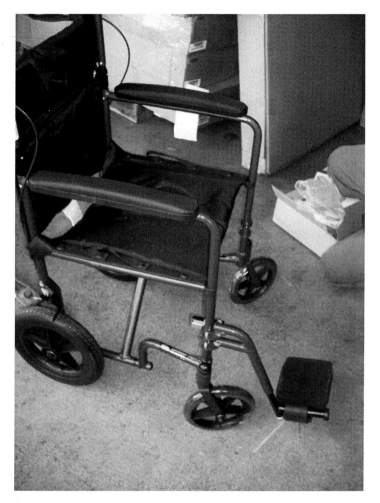

A transport, or "travel," wheelchair is designed to allow for easier community access and is much lighter than a standard manual wheelchair. This is an advantage for the caregiver who has to lift it into the trunk. The average weight is around 18 to 22 pounds. The transport wheelchair is not designed to be an everyday wheelchair if a care-receiver is a full-time wheelchair user. The transport wheelchair has four small wheels and is not designed for self-propulsion.

Reclining wheelchair

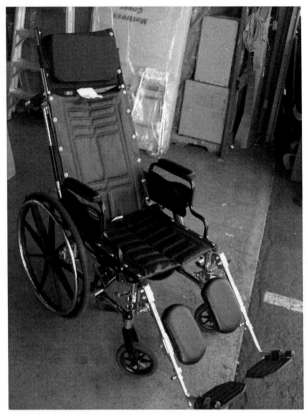

A reclining wheelchair has a seat back that reclines from a ver-
tical to a horizontal position and can be locked into the various
positions of recline. This type of wheelchair may be an appropriate
option for a care-receiver who requires more support and who has
difficulty with sitting upright due to weakness or low blood pressure. One problem with this type of chair, however, is that when the
back is reclined, it changes the hip angle in the seat, and care-receivers can slide down the chair and require frequent repositioning. This
type of chair is not ideal for the very dependent care-receiver or the
care-receiver who cannot weight-shift himself for pressure relief. In
such a case, a tilt-in-space wheelchair is a better option.

Tilt-in-space wheelchair

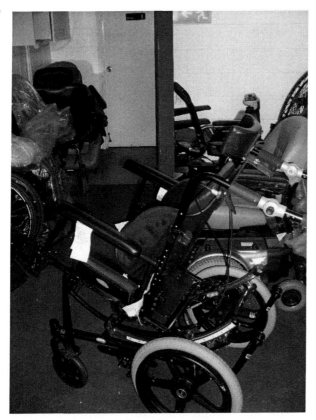

The tilt-in-space wheelchair is designed to tilt backward without changing the seat angle or the position of the care-receiver in the seat. This type of chair is a good option for care-receivers who are dependent on the wheelchair for all mobility and who may be at risk for skin breakdown in the buttocks due to immobility and decreased sensation. By tilting back the wheelchair, the weight is redistributed from the butt bones (ischial tuberosities, sacrum, and coccyx) to the back, allowing the blood to flow and nourish the skin. The effect of gravity on the spine in an upright sitting position is alleviated, causing less stress on the spine and the muscles, often resulting in increased sitting tolerance for a dependent care-receiver.

Medicare and Insurance Guidelines for Wheelchairs

Medicare and most major medical plans cover mobility devices, such as manual wheelchairs, power wheelchairs, and scooters. Typically, these insurers cover the least costly alternative that will meet the needs of the care-receiver. The Medicare guidelines change periodically but are available online and by request from the local Medicare offices. Durable medical equipment (DME) suppliers also should be able to provide these guidelines. Because the cost of different types of wheelchairs varies greatly, Medicare has assigned wheelchairs to different classes, based on function and need. Below is a general overview of the different classes, organized and titled by Medicare, for self-propelled manual wheelchair frames, as well as general requirements for reimbursement.

Standard wheelchair. This is the basic institutional wheelchair. There are no frame adjustments or modifications in this class. The wheelchair of steel-frame construction and generally weighs approximately 36 pounds, without the front riggings (leg rests). Size options are limited in this class as well. Seat-to-floor height is 19 to 21 inches.

> Appropriate clients: The care-receiver is typically able to propel a standard-weight wheelchair and does not require any special seating needs. He also does not require any modifications or atypical dimensions in the frame to self-propel the wheelchair or to perform transfers in and out of the wheelchair.

Standard hemi-wheelchair. This is the same class as the standard wheelchair, with the exception of having a lower seat-to-floor height and shorter footplate extension tubes. The seat-to-floor height in this category is typically 17 to 18 inches, which is low enough for foot propulsion for many care-receivers.

Appropriate clients: The care-receiver is of shorter physical stature or needs a lower seat-to-floor height to use his or her feet for propulsion.

Lightweight wheelchair. This class has more sizes available but is still limited. The standard seat width is 16 or 18 inches, but most chairs in this class are available with a 20-inch seat width and an 18-inch seat depth. There are few, if any, frame modifications or adjustments in this class. More options and accessories are available but are still limited. These chairs weigh less than 36 pounds, without front riggings, with an average of about 28 pounds. This class has a standard seat-to-floor height range of 19 to 21 inches.

Appropriate clients: The care-receiver for this class may be unable to propel the weight of a standard wheelchair due to upper and/or lower extremity weakness, low endurance or cardiopulmonary issues, pain, spasticity, and/or decreased range of motion but is able to propel himself in a lightweight chair of this class. Care-receivers who are appropriate for this class don't have significant deformities or spasticity and typically do not have a condition that is progressive in nature—there is little adjustability to accommodate any type of change, whether a physical or functional change.

Heavy-duty lightweight wheelchair. This class has more sizes, options, and accessories, as well as minimal frame adjustments, including a minimal adjustable axle plate. The standard seat width is 14, 16, or 18 inches, but most chairs of this class are available in a 20-inch seat width and 18-inch seat depth. These chairs weigh less than 34 pounds, without front riggings, with an average of around 26 pounds. This class has greater seat-to-floor options with available dimensions of 17 to 21 inches.

Appropriate clients: The care-receiver for this class may be unable to propel the weight of a standard or lightweight wheelchair due to upper and/or lower extremity weakness, low endurance or cardiopulmonary issues, pain, spasticity, and/or decreased range of motion, but he is able to propel in a lightweight chair of this class. The body dimensions of the care-receiver may require chair dimensions and adjustability that are not found in the lightweight class, such as greater or lesser seat-to-floor height, and higher back height than standard due to poor balance, postural control, abnormal tone, and/or other orthopedic issues. As in the lightweight class, care-receivers who are appropriate for this class of wheelchair don't have significant deformities or spasticity and typically do not have a condition that is progressive in nature.

Custom lightweight and ultra-lightweight wheelchair. This class has more sizes, options, and accessories, as well as many frame styles and adjustments, including adjustable axle plates, folding and rigid options, modular options, and different suspensions. The axle plate can be adjusted to a greater extent, allowing for ultimate customization in the wheelchair setup, which also can aid in injury prevention. There is much more adjustment in the caster housing, with greater options for angle of the seat. Greater options in caster sizes allow them to be tailored for the user. For example, micro-size castors can be used for a much tighter turning radius for sports or tight work areas, or wider casters can accommodate more difficult terrain. These chairs offer adjustable back angles to accommodate for lack of hip flexion. This class has more back-height options—low, medium, and tall.

The standard seat width is 14, 16, or 18 inches, but most chairs of this class are available with a 20-inch seat width and 18-inch seat depth. These chairs weigh less than 30 pounds, without front riggings, and may weigh as little as 17 to 18 pounds with a titanium frame. This class has greater seat-to-floor options, with available dimensions of 17 to 21 inches. This class of chair is more expensive and usually requires meticulous documentation and clear rationale for coverage by third-party payers.

Appropriate clients: This class has some of the same advantages of the heavy-duty lightweight class, with the added benefit of a much lighter wheelchair with a wide range of adjustments that may allow for greater accommodation of deformities and for greater independence on all terrains. Due to the adjustability, this class of wheelchair is the most appropriate of the manual wheelchairs for care-receivers with dynamic and/or progressive disorders. This class of chair requires much documentation by the physician or physical or occupational therapist. Basically, these wheelchairs are more expensive, and each component that increases the cost requires medical justification if it is to be covered by the insurance.

Motorized Wheelchairs and Scooters

Like the manual wheelchairs, power wheelchairs offer a vast number of options and features. Power wheelchair components can be even more complicated than manual. If the care-receiver has any needs that are greater than basic power mobility, it would be wise to consult with a physical or occupational therapist who is trained in this area and who can assist in making recommendations.

Scooters. Scooters are probably the simplest form of powered mobility. Scooters are controlled by a tiller that has a lever on the handle that controls speed and direction. Scooters take more energy to drive than driving a power wheelchair with a joystick control. Scooters also require, for the most part, use of two arms and relatively normal shoulder strength and range of motion. The care-receiver also will need to have at least fair strength in his hands to operate the controls. Scooters typically have a longer base than most power wheelchairs and therefore require a greater turning radius. In general, scooters are less costly, require greater gross arm strength, and have less accessibility indoors than a motorized wheelchair.

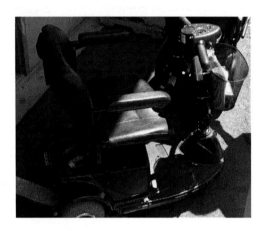

Motorized wheelchair. Motorized wheelchairs make use of either gears or belts, or sometimes both. Motorized wheelchairs with belt drives are typically very quiet, but they require more maintenance. Modern gear drives are fairly quiet and low-maintenance, but they tend to wear out more quickly than belt drives, and they get noisier in the process. Motorized wheelchairs vary in ruggedness. Low-end motorized wheelchairs have light frames that are suitable for indoor use, but when they are used to excess in the outdoors, the frames crack, front forks bend, and motors die. The latest high-priced electric wheelchairs are more rugged and reliable, with frames designed to handle more weight. Some newer electric models even have spring suspension, which allows a smooth ride over uneven territory.

Like the manual wheelchairs, there are many options available for motorized wheelchairs. If the care-receiver has special needs—such as needing alternative control devices because he may not have the arm and hand function to operate the wheelchair, or if he has spinal deformities that need to be accommodated—seek an evaluation from a qualified physical or occupational therapist to ensure the care-receiver gets the most appropriate equipment.

The type of motorized base can have a huge impact on accessibility within the home, so it's important to understand the differences.

Rear-wheel–drive wheelchairs are the traditional and most popular style. They generally are faster than front-wheel models but have poor turning capabilities as compared to front-wheel and mid-wheel models. **Front-wheel–drive wheelchairs** have become more common because they provide tighter turning functions. Most front-wheel–drive wheelchairs, however, have a slightly lower top speed than rear-wheel models because they tend to turn too readily at high speeds. **Mid-wheel–drive wheelchairs** provide the tightest turning of all because the wheelchair basically spins on itself, rather than turning wide, like the traditional rear-wheel model. The mid-wheel–drive is a good option for tight indoor spaces.

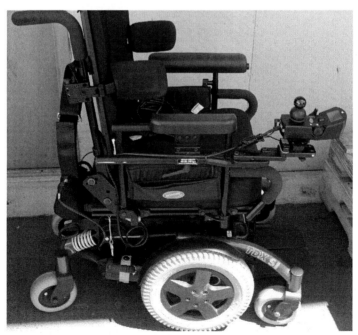

Mid-wheel–drive wheelchair

Additional wheelchair features that are available include:

- Electric wheelchair power tilt, a feature that tilts the entire seat assembly and footrests upward to a 45-degree angle
- Electric wheelchair recliner, a feature that tilts the seat back and raises the leg rests up horizontally.

Both of these features provide pressure relief and help to prevent pressure sores. If the care-receiver is unable to weight-shift or move around in the seat of the wheelchair, then excessive pressure can occur on the butt bones, which can lead to skin breakdown due to lack of blood circulation to that area. A power tilt allows for the weight to be distributed more to the back, allowing for the blood to nourish the skin under the butt bones to prevent skin breakdown.

CHAPTER TEN:

PASSIVE RANGE OF MOTION (PROM) EXERCISES

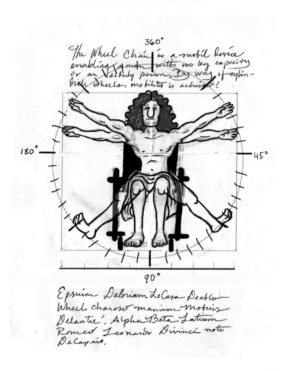

Passive range-of-motion (PROM) exercises are done *for* a care-receiver. As the caregiver, you perform these exercises because the care-receiver cannot do them by herself. PROM exercises may be needed, for example, if the care-receiver presents with paraplegia, quadriplegia, or hemiparesis. These conditions may be the result of a stroke, spinal cord injury, or head injury, or due to an array of diseases, such as multiple sclerosis or ALS. Range-of-motion exercises are particularly important if the care-receiver has to stay in bed or in a wheelchair. Without these exercises, joints, such as the knees and elbows, could become stiff and locked or get stuck in a shortened position (called a contracture). Contractures in joints can cause pain or limit the ability for dressing and hygiene. PROM exercises help keep joint areas flexible but do not build up muscles or make them stronger. The arm exercises can be performed in a chair or bed. The leg exercises are best performed with the care-receiver lying flat on his back in bed.

How to Perform PROM Exercises

As the caregiver, you will move the care-receiver's limb or joint through its available range of motion (ROM) and hold it in this stretched or elongated position for at least twenty seconds. The longer the hold, the better, as the goal is to maintain or increase the resting length of the muscle tissue and tendons. The movement should always be slow and sustained. This is especially important if the care-receiver has spasticity, which is constant muscle spasms (tightening). If the movement is fast, the spasticity or muscle tension will actually increase, making it even harder to move the limb. By going slowly, you can, in a way, "sneak up" on the spasticity and be less likely to set it off or make it stronger. Spasticity is often seen in care-receivers who have suffered a stroke, head injury, or spinal cord injury, as well as in those who have cerebral palsy or multiple sclerosis. The care-receiver may feel a slight discomfort when the joint is moved through the full range of motion, due to the stretching of the muscle. Mild discomfort may be expected, but stop the passive range-of-motion exercises if the care-receiver feels pain. (Watch for signs of pain if the care-receiver is non-verbal.) The exercises should never cause pain or go beyond the normal movement of the joint. If there is any doubt about how to perform these exercises, ask the care-receiver's physician for a referral to physical or occupational therapy for proper instruction. If the care-receiver cannot move his limbs or head, PROM exercises need to be part of the daily routine to avoid contractures.

Use good posture while performing PROM exercises for your care-receiver. Standing, or sitting as straight as possible, will protect your back. Keep your normal lumbar curve (as mentioned in chapter one) to avoid stress or injury.

The following PROM exercises are organized by body part:

Neck Exercises

Neck rotation. Turn the care-receiver's head toward the right, as if he were looking over his right shoulder. Then slowly turn his head so that he is looking over his left shoulder. The head is turned only far enough so that the care-receiver's nose lines up above his shoulder.

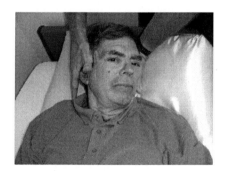 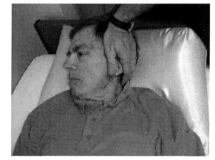

Head tilts. Cup your hands behind the care-receiver's head, with your thumbs around each side of the head. Tilt the care-receiver's head to the side, bringing the right ear toward the right shoulder. Then slowly tilt her head to bring the left ear toward the left shoulder.

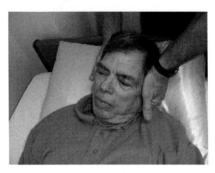

Shoulder and Elbow Exercises

Shoulder flexion (reaching motion in front of the body). Place one hand under the care-receiver's elbow, and hold her wrist with the other hand. With the care-receiver's elbow straight (in extension), lift her arm straight up and back so that her elbow is as close as possible to her ear.

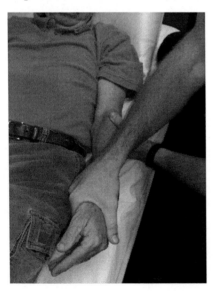
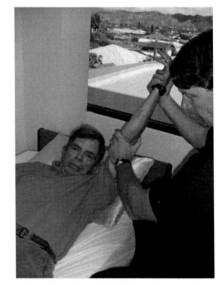

Shoulder abduction (moving arm away from side). Place one hand under the care-receiver's elbow, and hold his wrist with the other hand. With the care-receiver's elbow straight (in extension), bring his arm up from the side of his body and as close to his ear as possible.

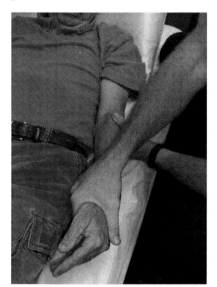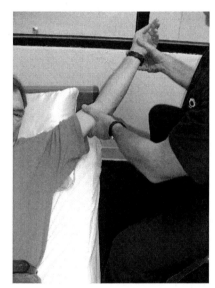

Shoulder abduction

Shoulder external rotation. The care-receiver should be positioned lying flat on her back on the bed. With the care-receiver's elbow bent to 90 degrees and positioned at the same level as the shoulder, slowly rotate her arm backward so that the back of her forearm and hand are as close as possible to the bed.

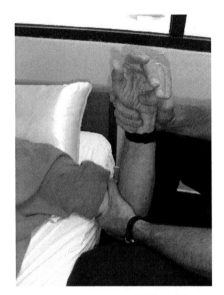
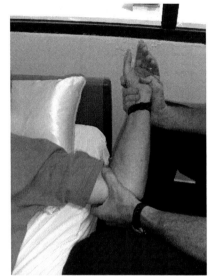

Shoulder external rotation

Elbow flexion and extension. With the care-receiver's right arm at his side, turn his hand so that it is palm up. Then bend the arm at the elbow so that the care-receiver's fingers point toward the ceiling, and continue bending the elbow until the fingertips touch the front of the right shoulder.

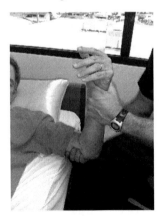
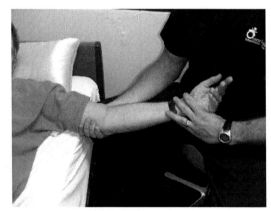

Elbow flexion and extension

Wrist Exercises: These exercises can be performed while sitting or in bed.

Wrist flexion and extension. Hold the care-receiver's wrist and hand, with her palm facing down, and bend the hand back and forward through the available range of motion.

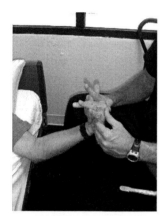 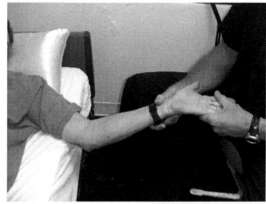

Forearm supination and pronation (palm up, palm down). With the care-receiver's elbow and forearm on the bed, raise her hand and gently twist so that the palm of the hand faces up and then down.

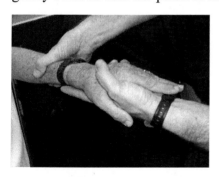 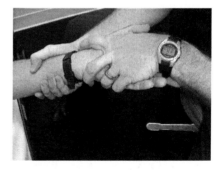

Hand and Finger Exercises

Hold the care-receiver's wrist to keep it straight. Use your other hand to do the hand and finger exercises.

Finger flexion and extension. Place your hand on the back of the care-receiver's fingers and gently bend his hand into a fist; then straighten the fingers again.

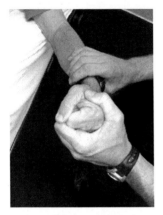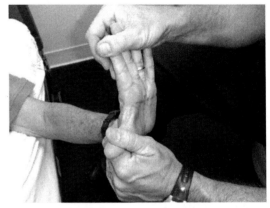

Finger spreads. Straighten out the care-receiver's fingers, and spreads the fingers wide apart, one at a time.

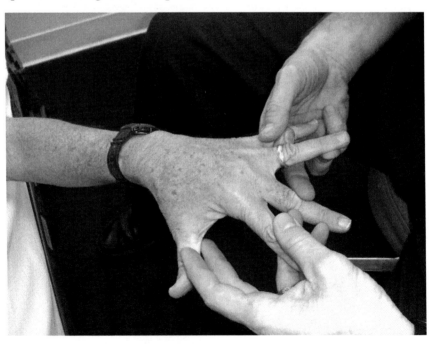

Hip and Knee Exercises

If the care-receiver has had a hip injury or surgery, do hip exercises only with instructions from a physician or physical therapist. Total hip replacement precautions do not allow for the following motions:

1. Hip flexion past 90 degrees
2. Hip adduction or leg crossing midline
3. Hip rotation or toes pointing inward

Hip and knee flexion and extension. With one hand under the care-receiver's thigh and the other hand under his calf, slowly bend the hip and knee up toward the chest as much as possible.

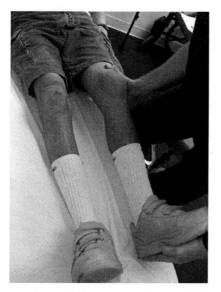 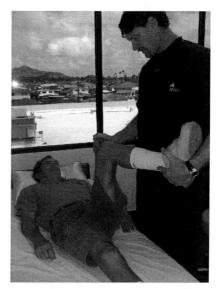

Hip abduction (side to side). Move the care-receiver's leg out to the side as far as possible, and then return the leg to the start position (see picture at top of next page).

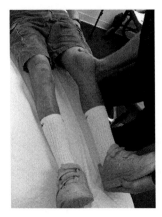
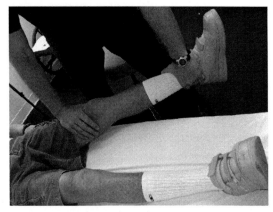

Hip rotation (in and out). Bend the care-receiver's knee so the bottom of the right foot is flat on the bed. While keeping the knee bent and the foot in contact with the bed, roll the leg inward as far as possible, and try to touch the bed with the big toe; then roll the leg outward as far as possible and try to touch the bed with the small toe.

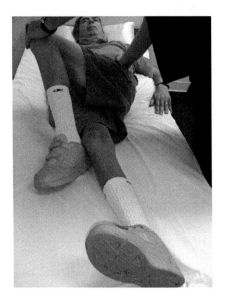

Ankle Exercises

Ankle dorsiflexion (bends). Take hold of the care-receiver's heel with one hand and pull the heel bone. At the same time, push his foot with your forearm (using the same arm). Push the foot until the toes are in the direction of the care-receiver's head.

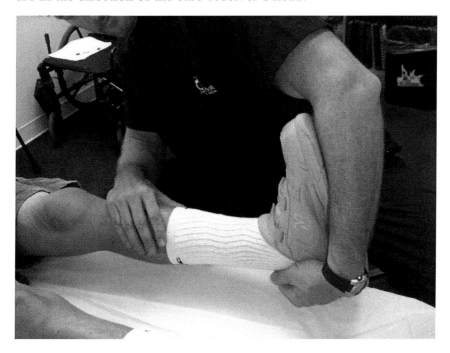

CHAPTER ELEVEN:

SEATED AND BED-LEVEL EXERCISES

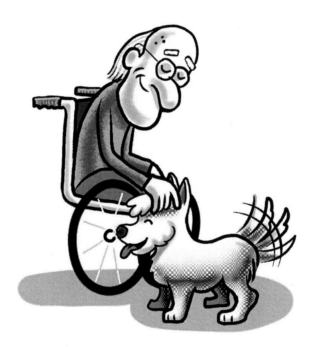

Exercise is an important element that should be a part of everyone's daily routine, especially seniors—this includes both the caregiver and the care-receiver. Physical activity and exercise is one way to maintain health and mobility. Often, the care-receiver will be given a home exercise program by physicians or a physical or occupational therapist, and the caregiver will be responsible for helping the care-receiver to carry out the program.

The exercises presented here are divided into three routines based on the level of mobility and capability of the care-receiver. As the caregiver, you can choose the level that best fits your care-receiver's (and your own) mobility profile.

Level One: Moderate to Severe Symptomatic (wheelchair or walking with walker, with assistance)

This group of exercises is appropriate for anyone because they do not require balance in stance. They are especially appropriate for anyone who is wheelchair-bound or who uses an assistive device that requires bilateral upper-extremity support, such as a walker. The exercises in this category are primarily performed while sitting or lying down. The recommendation is to start out with one set of ten repetitions for each exercise and build up to performing two to three sets of ten, as tolerated. When starting out, you and the care-receiver can break up the exercises, performing them on different days so as not to perform a large volume of exercises at one time. For example, alternate performing the sitting exercise with the mat exercises. A good schedule would be to perform the sitting group on Monday, Wednesday, Friday and the mat exercise group on Tuesday and Thursdays. In general, it is best to limit exercise time to twenty to thirty minutes, maximum, per exercise session. Try to get into the habit of exercising daily for fifteen or twenty minutes, rather than skipping days and then trying to "make up" for missing days. If the exercises in the suggested list below cannot be completed in one session, complete the group of exercises on the next day. Again, the main point is to exercise daily.

Suggested Exercise List

Sitting exercise routine
1. Static wall sitting
2. Wall sitting arm raise
3. Wall sitting arm diagonals
4. Wall sitting alternate leg lifts
5. Wall sitting alternate arm/leg lifts
6. Wood chop

Mat/bed exercise routine
1. Bridges
2. Lower trunk rotation
3. Alternating leg lifts
4. Alternating arm/leg lifts

Sitting Wall Exercises

The sitting wall exercises are appropriate for those who are wheel-chair-bound or who use assistive devices that require bilateral upper-extremity support, such as a walker. The emphasis is on promoting an erect posture. The contact with the wall acts as a guide and gives the postural muscles feedback. It may feel like someone is behind, pushing forward, as the upper and lower back muscles may not be accustomed to holding the back straight. The goal is to retrain these muscles to maintain a more erect posture so that the skeletal system will be more mechanically stacked; it then requires less energy to maintain an upright posture.

Wall sitting

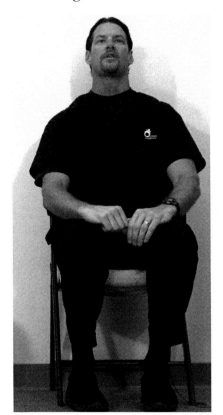 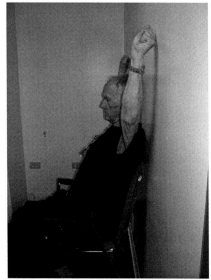

Beginner Level

EXERCISE POSITION: Sit with buttocks completely at back of a chair, with shoulders and head against wall and with arms up. Hold posture for thirty seconds.

Wall sitting arm raise

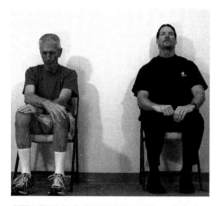 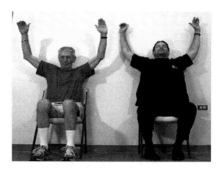

START POSITION: Sit with buttocks all the way back in the chair, with shoulders and head against the wall. Bring up the arms to where the elbows are the same level as the shoulders, with the elbow bent to 90 degrees. Maintain as much contact of arms with the wall as possible.

ACTION/FINISH POSITION: Pinch the shoulder blades together and maintain full contact with the wall. Slowly raise the arms over the head until the elbows are completely straight. Hold this position for ten seconds, and slowly return to start position.

Wall sitting alternating leg lifts

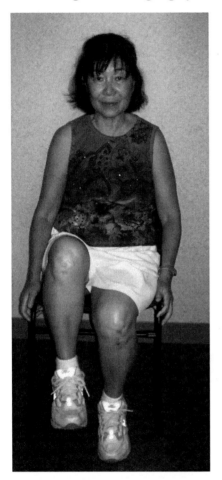 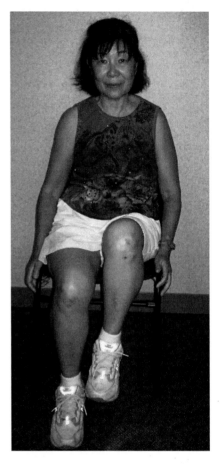

START POSITION: Sit with buttocks as far back in the chair as possible, with the shoulders and head against the wall.

ACTION/FINISH POSITION: While maintaining contact with the wall, shift weight to the right leg and lift the left leg, as if marching. Return to starting position and repeat with the opposite side; continue by lifting alternate legs.

Wall sitting alternating arm/leg lifts

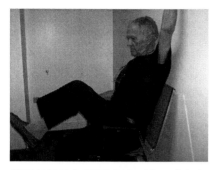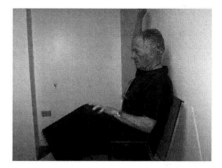

START POSITION: Sit with buttocks as far back in chair as possible, with shoulders and head against wall.

ACTION/FINISH POSITION: While maintaining contact with the wall, shift weight to the right leg and lift the left leg, while simultaneously raising the right arm. Return to starting position and perform on opposite side, and repeat by lifting the opposite arm/leg.

Wall sitting arm diagonals

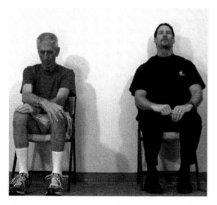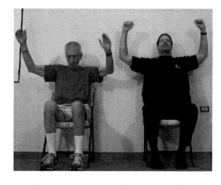

START POSITION: Sit with buttocks as far back as possible in chair, with shoulders and head against wall and with hands over opposite hip, such as the right hand over the left hip and the left hand over the right hip.

ACTION/FINISH POSITION: Maintain contact with the wall during the exercise. Pinch the shoulder blades together while lifting the arms simultaneously in a diagonal position, until the arms are over the head, with elbows extended.

Wood chop

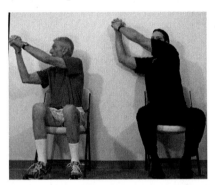 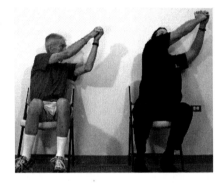

START POSITION: Sit with buttocks as far back as possible in chair, with shoulders and head against wall. Grasp hands together and place on outside of one knee.

ACTION/FINISH POSITION: Lift the arms from the outside of the knee up toward and over the opposite shoulder, while rotating the upper trunk in the same direction as the hands. Return the hands to the lap, and repeat motion to other side.

Mat Exercises

Mat exercises do not require the ability to balance and are appropriate for anyone, as long as the required positions can be achieved. The exercises that may be the most difficult are those with positions that require lying on the stomach. The focus of mat exercises is the same as with the wall exercises—to strengthen the postural muscles and promote good posture.

Supine (lying on back)

Bridges full arm contact

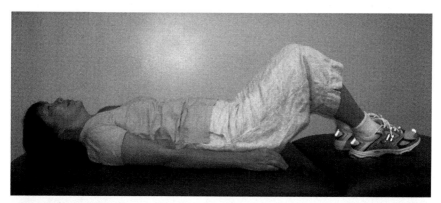

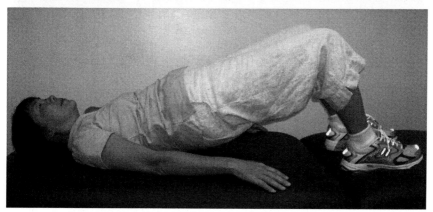

START POSITION: Lie down on the back with the arms straight down by the side. Bend both of the knees to where the feet are flat on the mat or bed.

ACTION/FINISH POSITION: Hold the stomach tight and squeeze the buttocks muscles, while lifting the buttocks as high off the mat or bed as possible. Hold the bridge position for five seconds, and return to starting position.

Alternate arm positions for bridges (more challenging)

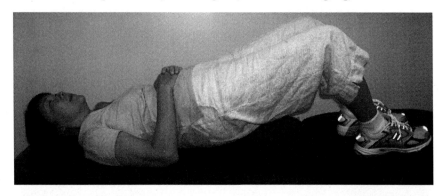

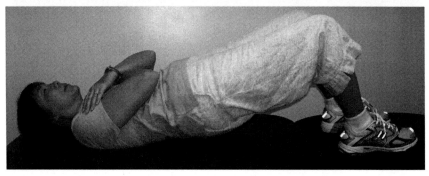

START POSITION: Lie on the back with the elbows in contact with the bed or mat and with arms resting on stomach or crossed on chest. These alternate arm positions lessen the contact of the upper extremities with the bed or floor, making the exercise more challenging. Bend both of the knees to where the feet are flat on the mat or bed.

ACTION/FINISH POSITION: Hold the stomach tight while squeezing the buttocks muscles. Lift the buttocks as high off the mat or bed as possible. Hold the bridge position for five seconds, and return to starting position.

Bridges alternate leg lift

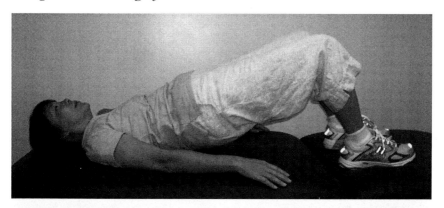

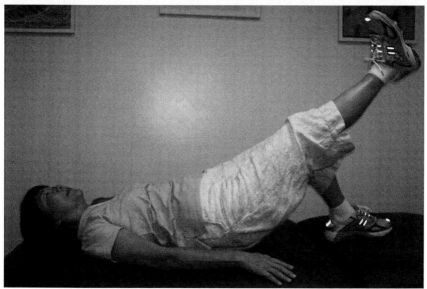

START POSITION: Lie on back with the arms straight down by the side. Bend both of the knees to where the feet are flat on the mat or bed.

ACTION/FINISH POSITION: Hold the stomach tight while squeezing the buttocks muscles. Lift the buttocks as high off the mat or bed as possible. Hold the bridge position while extending the right leg, and hold for five seconds. While still maintaining the bridge, return the right leg to the mat and repeat on left side, while maintaining the bridge. Return to starting position, and then repeat for the desired number of repetitions.

Lower trunk rotation (windshield washers)

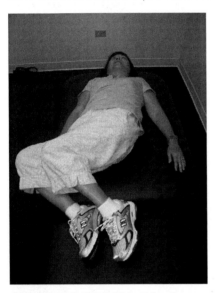 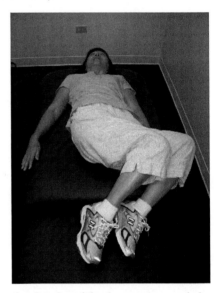

START POSITION: Lie down on the back with the arms straight down by the side. Bend both of the knees to where the feet are flat on the mat or bed.

ACTION/FINISH POSITION: Maintain the shoulders in contact with the bed during the entire exercise. While keeping the knees and feet together, roll the knees as far to the right as possible (may feel a stretch on the opposite side). Hold for three seconds, and then roll the knees as far as possible to the left side. Return to starting position, and then repeat for the desired number of repetitions.

Alternating leg lifts

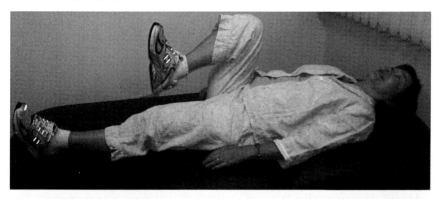

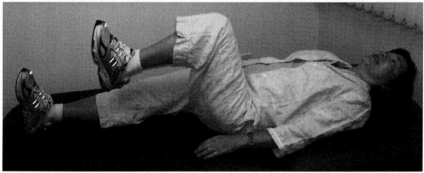

Beginner Level

START POSITION: Lie flat with arms down to side and legs extended.

ACTION/FINISH POSITION: While maintaining contact with the mat or bed, shift weight to the right leg and lift the left leg, as if marching, while lying down. Return to starting position and perform on opposite side; continue by alternately lifting the legs.

Alternating arm/leg lifts

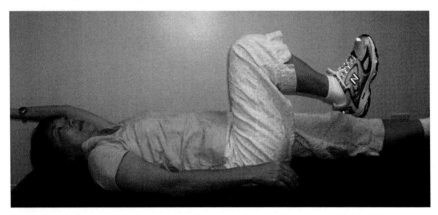

START POSITION: Lie flat with arms down to side and legs extended.

ACTION/FINISH POSITION: While maintaining contact with the mat or bed, shift weight to the right leg and lift the left leg, as if marching, while lying down and concurrently raising the opposite arm over your head. Return to starting position and perform on opposite side; continue by alternately lifting the arm with the opposite leg.

PURPOSE: This exercise stimulates and works the postural muscles as weight shifts to off-load the opposite leg. It promotes a more normal gait with arm swing.

CHAPTER TWELVE:

STANDING AND BED-LEVEL EXERCISES FOR MINIMALLY TO MODERATELY PHYSICALLY IMPAIRED

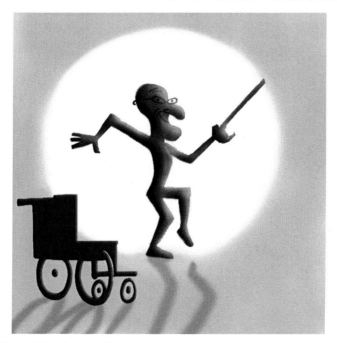

Level Two: Moderate Symptomatic (impaired balance; requires assistive device)

This group of exercises is good for those with minimal to moderately impaired balance. These exercises may require more complex movements that involve greater coordination than the simpler exercises presented in chapter eleven. If there is a history of falling and/or use of an assistive device that requires just one hand, such as a cane, these exercises are appropriate. The more advanced leg and balance exercises can be modified by using some support of the arms for safety. If balance is impaired to the level that it does not allow for safe performance of the exercises while standing, please use the sitting and mat exercises in chapter eleven. The emphasis is on promoting an erect posture. The contact with the wall gives the postural muscles feedback and acts as a guide. By retraining the postural muscles to maintain a more erect posture, the skeletal system will be more mechanically stacked; less energy is then required to maintain an upright position.

Suggested Exercise List

Modified standing exercise routine
1. Static wall standing with chair
2. Wall standing arm raise
3. Wall standing arm diagonals
4. Wall squats with chair

Mat/bed exercise routine
1. Bridges
2. Lower trunk rotation
3. Superman
4. Airplane

Standing Wall Exercises
The standing exercises in this category require the ability for general balance, with or without the need for upper-extremity support. If balance is impaired to the level that it does not allow for safe performance of the standing exercises, please go back to the sitting and mat exercises in chapter eleven.

Static wall standing
EXERCISE POSITION: Stand with heels, buttocks, shoulders and head against wall and hold posture for thirty seconds.

EXERCISE MODIFICATION FOR DECREASED BALANCE: The above exercise can also be performed with a walker or tall-back chair (turned around) for greater balance in standing if needed. Try to minimize the weight-bearing through the arms so that the balance can be challenged safely.

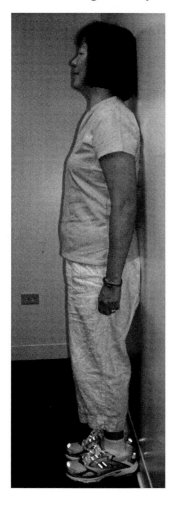 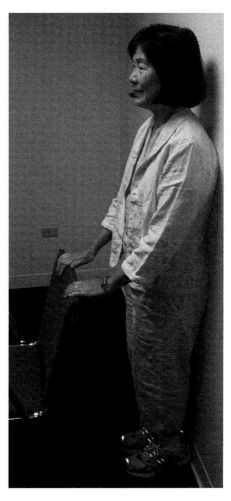

Wall standing arm raise

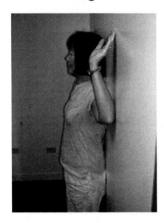 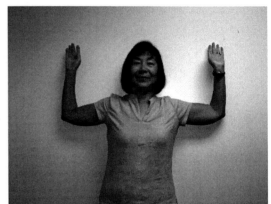

START POSITION: Stand with heels, buttocks, shoulders, and head against wall. Bring up the arms to where the elbow is the same level as the shoulder, with elbow bent to 90 degrees. Arms should maintain as much contact with the wall as possible.

ACTION/FINISH POSITION: Pinch the shoulder blades together and maintain full contact with the wall, while slowly raising the arms over the head until the elbows are completely straight. Hold this position for ten seconds, and slowly return back to start position.

Wall standing alternate leg lift

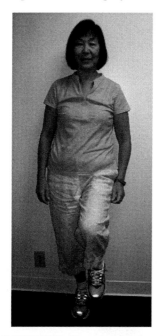 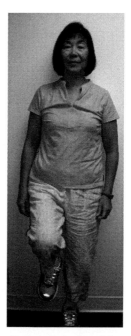

START POSITION: Stand with heels, buttocks, shoulders, and head against wall.

ACTION/FINISH POSITION: While maintaining contact with the wall, purposely shift weight to the right leg, and lift the left leg. Return to starting position and perform on opposite side; continue by alternately lifting the legs.

EXERCISE MODIFICATION FOR DECREASED BALANCE: The above exercise can also be performed with a walker or tall-back chair (turned around) for greater balance in standing, if needed. Try to minimize the weight-bearing through the arms so that the balance can be challenged safely.

Wall standing diagonals

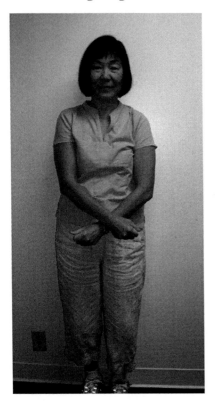 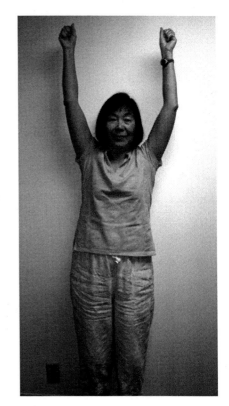

Intermediate Level

START POSITION: Stand with heels, buttocks, shoulders, and head against wall, with hands over opposite hip, such as left hand over the right hip, and right hand over the left hip.

ACTION/FINISH POSITION: Maintain contact with the wall during the exercise. Pinch the shoulder blades together, while lifting the arms simultaneously in a diagonal position until the arms are over the head, with elbows extended.

Wall standing squats

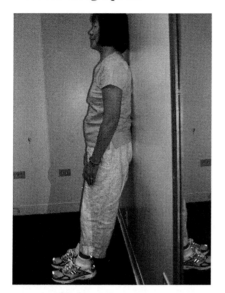 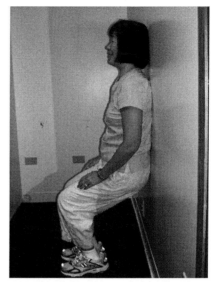

START POSITION: Stand with heels approximately 18 inches from the wall, with buttocks, shoulders, and head against wall.

ACTION/FINISH POSITION: Buttocks, shoulders, and head should maintain contact with the wall, while sliding down and up the wall. The bottom of the squat position will be dictated by the available strength in the legs. Do not squat deeper than 90 degrees at the hip, which is when the hip and knees are at the same level. The deeper the squat, the greater the strength that is required. A modification for this exercise is to place the feet farther away from the wall, which decreases weight-bearing and makes the exercise easier.

Mat Exercises

The mat exercises do not require much balance and are appropriate for anyone, as long as the required positions can be achieved. The exercises that may be the most difficult to achieve are those with positions that require lying on the stomach. The focus of mat exercises is the same as the wall exercises, which is to strengthen the postural muscles to better combat the forward posturing.

Supine (lying on back)

Bridges

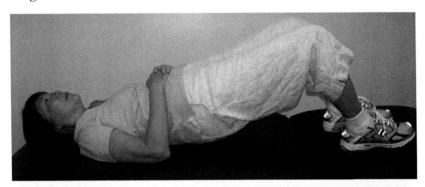

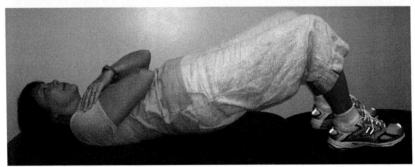

START POSITION: Lie down on the back with the elbows in contact with the bed or mat and arms resting on stomach, or with arms crossed on chest. These alternate arm positions lessen the contact of the upper extremities with the bed or floor, which makes the exercise more challenging. Bend both of the knees to where the feet are flat on the mat or bed.

ACTION/FINISH POSITION: Hold the stomach tight while squeezing the buttocks muscles. Lift the buttocks as high off the mat or bed as possible. Hold the bridge position for five seconds, and return to starting position.

Lower trunk rotation (windshield washers)

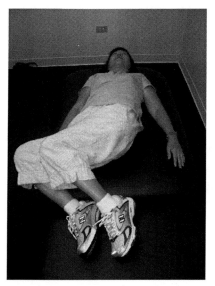 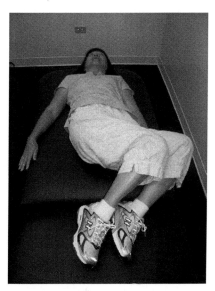

Beginner Level

START POSITION: Lie on the back with arms straight down on the side of the body. Bend both of the knees to where the feet are flat on the mat or bed.

ACTION/FINISH POSITION: Shoulders should maintain contact with the bed during the entire exercise. While keeping the knees and feet together, roll the knees as far to the right as possible. Hold for three seconds, and then roll the knees as far as possible to the left side. Return to starting position, and then repeat for the desired number of repetitions.

Superman

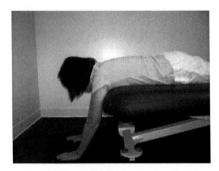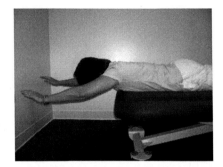

START POSITION: Lie flat on the stomach with the arms hanging down over the front edge of the mat or bed.

ACTION/FINISH POSITION: Lift the arms straight up in front of the body in approximately a 45-degree angle. The position will look like Superman's arms when he is flying. Hold this position for five seconds, and repeat to complete the desired number of repetitions. Keep the head and neck neutral, with eyes looking straight down toward the floor. Do not look forward, which will hyper-extend the neck.

Airplane

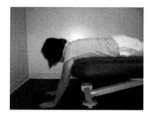 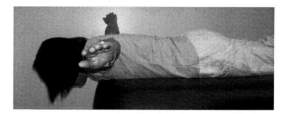

START POSITION: Lie flat on the stomach, with the arms hanging down over the side edge of the mat or bed.

ACTION/FINISH POSITION: Lift the arms out to the side as high as possible, with the wrist, elbow, and shoulders all in a line. The arm position will look like the wings of an airplane. Hold this position for five seconds, and repeat to complete the desired number of repetitions. Keep the head and neck neutral, with the eyes looking straight down to the floor. Do not look forward, which will hyperextend the neck.

CHAPTER THIRTEEN:

STANDING AND BED-LEVEL EXERCISES FOR MINIMALLY PHYSICALLY IMPAIRED

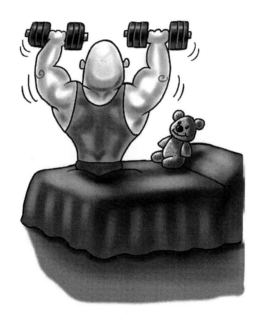

Level Three: Mildly Symptomatic (good standing balance, no assistive device)

This group of exercises will require the ability for good general balance, without the need for upper-extremity support. If balance is impaired to the level that it does not allow for safe performance of the standing exercises, please go back to the Level Two exercise program in chapter twelve. The recommendation is to start out with one set of ten repetitions for each exercise, and build up to performing two to three sets of ten, as tolerated.

Suggested Exercise List:

Standing exercise routine

1. Wall standing arm raise

2. Wall standing arm diagonals

3. Wall standing alternate arm/leg lift

4. Standing squats

5. Lunges

Mat/bed exercise routine

1. Bridges with leg lifts

2. Lower trunk rotation

3. Superman

4. Airplane

5. Alternating arm/leg lifts on stomach

Standing Wall Exercises

The standing exercises require the ability for general balance without the need for upper-extremity support.

Wall standing arm raise

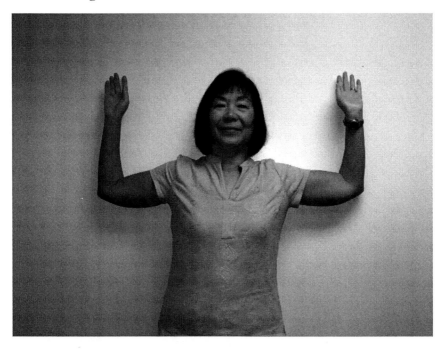

START POSITION: Stand with heels, buttocks, shoulders, and head against wall. Bring up the arms to where the elbow is the same level as the shoulder, with the elbow bent to 90 degrees. Arms should maintain as much contact with the wall as possible.

ACTION/FINISH POSITION: Pinch the shoulder blades together, and maintain full contact with the wall. Slowly raise the arms over the head until the elbows are completely straight. Hold this position for ten seconds, and slowly return back to start position.

Wall standing diagonals

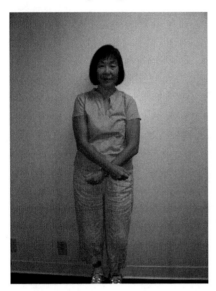 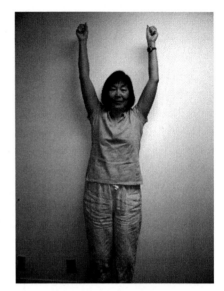

START POSITION: Stand with heels, buttocks, shoulders, and head against wall, with hands over opposite hip, such as right hand over left hip, and left hand over right hip.

ACTION/FINISH POSITION: Maintaining contact with the wall during the exercise. Pinch the shoulder blades together, while lifting the arms simultaneously in a diagonal position, until the arms are over the head with elbows extended.

Wall standing alternating arm/leg lift

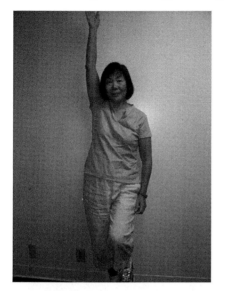 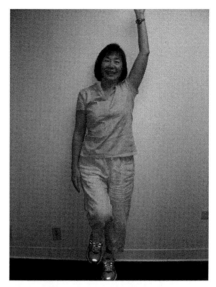

START POSITION: Stand with heels, buttocks, shoulders, and head against wall.

ACTION/FINISH POSITION: While maintaining contact with the wall, purposely shift weight to the right leg and lift the left leg, while simultaneously raising the right arm. Return to starting position and perform to opposite side, and repeat by alternating lifting the opposite arm/leg.

Standing squats

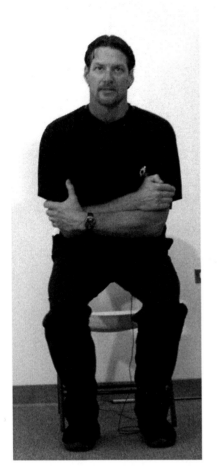 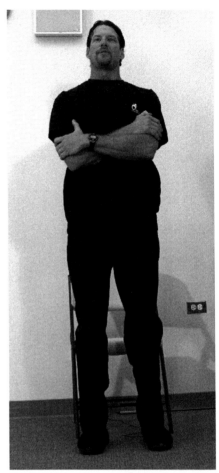

START POSITION; ACTION/FINISH POSITION: From sitting, scoot forward from a chair or bed so that the feet are flat on the floor. Fold the arms across the chest. Bend forward at the hip, while keeping the back straight. Keep bending forward until the nose is past the toes. Straighten out the legs into standing. Reverse the motion to sit down (in a controlled manner, not falling back into the chair). If this is too difficult, push with the arms to initiate standing, and use the arms on the thighs to lower back into the chair or bed.

Standing lunges

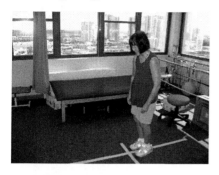 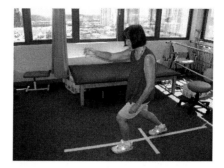

START POSITION: Stand with a less than shoulder-width base of support, with the toes even.

ACTION/FINISH POSITION: Lunge forward with one leg, while keeping opposite leg in its original position. Return to starting position, and repeat with opposite leg.

Mat Exercises

The focus of mat exercises is the same as for the wall exercises—to strengthen the postural muscles.

Bridges alternate leg lift

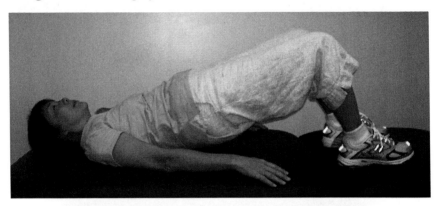

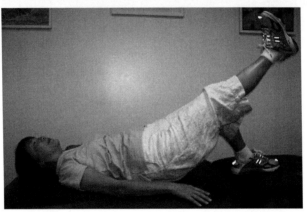

START POSITION: Lie down on the back with the arms straight down by the side of the body. Bend both of the knees to where the feet are flat on the mat or bed.

ACTION/FINISH POSITION: Hold the stomach tight, and squeeze the buttocks muscles. Lift the buttocks as high off the mat or bed as possible. Hold the bridge position while extending or straightening the right lower leg, and hold for five seconds.

The right and left thighs should be even, or parallel. While still maintaining the bridge position, return the right leg to the mat, and repeat on left side. Return to starting position, and then repeat for the desired number of repetitions.

PURPOSE: This exercise focuses on the postural muscles for hip and back extension, as well as core strengthening. The hip and back extensors will help to maintain the strength and motion for a more upright posture.

Lower trunk rotation (windshield washers)

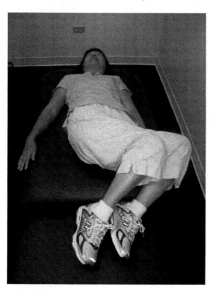 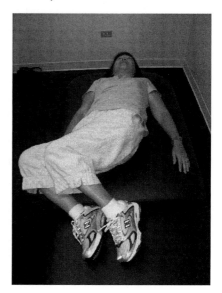

Beginner Level
START POSITION: Lie down on the back with the arms extended by the side. Bend both of the knees to where the feet are flat on the mat or bed.

ACTION/FINISH POSITION: Shoulders should maintain contact with the bed during the entire exercise. While keeping the knees and feet together, roll the knees as far to the right as possible. Hold for three seconds, and then roll the knees as far as possible to the left side. Return to starting position, and then repeat for the number amount of repetitions.

Superman

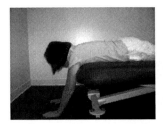 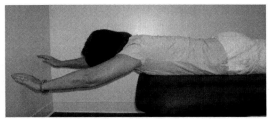

START POSITION: Lie flat on the stomach with the arms hanging down over the front edge of the mat or bed.

ACTION/FINISH POSITION: Lift the arms straight up in front of the body in approximately a 45-degree angle. The position will look like Superman's arms when he is flying. Hold this position for five seconds, and repeat to complete the desired number of repetitions. Keep the head and neck neutral, with your eyes looking straight down to the floor. Do not look forward, which will hyper-extend the neck.

Airplane

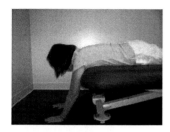 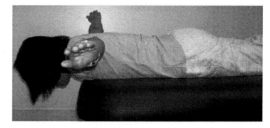

START POSITION: Lie flat on the stomach with the arms hanging down over the side edge of the mat or bed.

ACTION/FINISH POSITION: Lift your arms out to side as high as possible, with the wrist, elbow, and shoulders in line. The arm position will look like the wings of an airplane. Hold this position for five seconds, and repeat to complete the desired number of repetitions. Keep the head and neck neutral, with the eyes looking straight down. Do not look forward, which will hyper-extend the neck.

Alternate leg/arm lifts on stomach

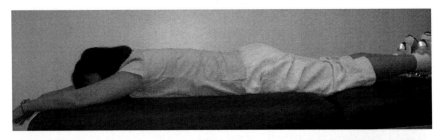

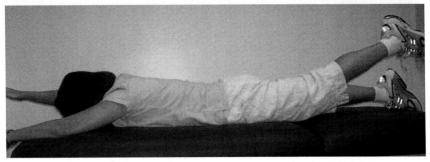

START POSITION: Lie flat on the stomach, with the arms and legs straight.

ACTION/FINISH POSITION: Purposely shift weight to the right leg and lift the left leg, while simultaneously raising the right arm. Return to starting position and perform on opposite side, and repeat by alternately lifting the opposite arm/leg.

GLOSSARY

active motion: Movement of a body part against gravity

cervical: Pertaining to the neck

contracture: Shortening of muscle or connective tissue that prevents a joint or muscle from moving through its full range of motion

dementia: Loss of brain function, mental confusion, decreased cognition

endurance: The ability of the muscle to execute repeated contractions

extension: The movement by which the two ends of any joint part draw away from each other

facet joints: The junction or articulation of two vertebrae (back bones). Movement of the back takes place at these joints.

flexion: The act of bending or moving the two ends of a joint part closer together or bending forward at the waist

hemiplegia/hemiparesis: Motor and/or sensory impairment on one side of the body

intravertebral disc: A structure located between two vertebrae of the spine that acts like a shock absorber

kyphosis: Abnormally increased curvature of the upper back; also referred to as "humping" or kyphotic posture

ligament: A band of fibrous tissue that connects bones or cartilage and thereby supports the joints

lumbar: Pertaining to the low back

neglect: Not attending to, recognizing, or acknowledging the affected side of the body

nerve root: Individual nerve as it exits from the spinal cord

neutral spine: Maintaining the normal spinal curves

occupational therapist: A licensed professional who works to restore the independence of clients in their daily life tasks after a physically disabling impairment

osteoarthritis: Degenerative joint disease occurring chiefly in older persons; characterized by degeneration of the joint surfaces

osteoporosis: A metabolic bone disease associated with loss of bone mass, even though the mineral content remains normal; loss of bone mass contributes to fractures, back pain, and deformities

Parkinson's disease: A slow-progressing neurological disorder characterized by slow movements, muscle rigidity, and tremors

passive range of motion: The movement of a person's muscles to a stretched position by someone else

physical therapist: A licensed professional who works to restore normal function in persons who have suffered a physically debilitating ailment and difficulties in mobility

postural hypotension: A drop in blood pressure when moving from a lying or sitting position to standing, which causes a lack of blood flow to the brain, with potential light-headedness

power: Maximal strength-producing capacity of an individual, expressed relative to time; Force x Distance/Time

pressure sores: A breakdown of skin and other tissues from continuous sitting or lying

quadriplegia: Neurological impairment in all four extremities and the trunk, with complete or incomplete damage to the spinal cord

range of motion: The degree of movement that a body part is able to accomplish

rigidity: Stiffness in muscles that causes internal resistance to movement; often seen in Parkinson's disease and characterized as "cog-wheel rigidity" due to a catch-and-release feel when attempting to move a limb

rounded back: A posture characterized by loss of normal lumbar (low back) curve

sciatica: Pain radiating down the sciatic nerve into the posterior (back part of) the thigh and leg

sensory: Relating to perception by senses (taste, touch, smell, sight, and hearing)

spasm: Sudden tightening of muscles

spasticity: An abnormal, velocity-dependent increase (the faster the limb is moved, the greater the spasticity) in muscle tone due to damage to the brain or spinal cord; spasticity can be present in individuals with closed head injury, stroke, spinal cord injury, multiple sclerosis, hereditary spastic paraparesis, and cerebral palsy.

squat pivot transfer: A type of transfer where the care-receiver can bear at least partial weight through his legs from a squatting position, with assist from a caregiver

strain: Overstress of a muscle to the extent that some internal injury occurs to the muscle fibers

standing pivot transfer: A type of transfer where the caregiver assists a care-receiver by helping him with balance and not with weight-bearing through his legs

strength: A muscle's ability to produce maximum force

swayback: A posture characterized by an excessive lumbar (low back) curve

tendon: Connective tissue that connects muscle to bone

thoracic: Pertaining to the part of the spine between the neck (cervical) and the lower back (lumbar); the upper back region

vertebrae: Bones that link together to form the spinal column

APPENDIX A

Caregiver Organizations

- **Children of Aging Parents (CAPS)**
  800-227-7294
  Website: www.caps4caregivers.org

CAPS assists caregivers of the elderly with information and referrals, a network of support groups, and publications and programs that promote public awareness of the value and the needs of family caregivers.

- **Family Caregiver Alliance (FCA)**
  800-445-8106
  Website: www.caregiver.org
  E-mail: info@caregiver.org

FCA is the leading agency in California's system of caregiver resource centers. FCA provides support and help to family caregivers and champions their cause through education, services, research, and advocacy. Services are specific to California, although information can be accessed nationally.

- **Family Voices, Inc.**
  888-835-5669
  Website: www.familyvoices.org

Family Voices offers information on health-care policies relevant to special-needs children in every state.

- **Friends' Health Connection**
  800-483-7436
  Website: www.48friend.org

Friends' Health Connection links persons with illness or disability and their family caregivers with others experiencing the same challenges.

- **National Alliance for Caregiving**
  Website: www.caregiving.org

Although not an organization that helps family caregivers directly, the National Alliance for Caregiving's website provides resources for family caregivers.

- **National Family Caregivers Association**
  800-896-3650
  Website: www.thefamilycaregiver.org
  E-mail: info@thefamilycaregiver.org

NFCA is a national nonprofit organization dedicated to empowering family caregivers to act on behalf of themselves and their loved ones, and to remove barriers to their health and well-being.

- **Rosalynn Carter Institute for Human Development (RCI)**
  229-928-1234
  Website: www.rci.gsw.edu

RCI provides educational programs for caregivers, conducts research, and disseminates information about caregiving.

- **U.S. Department of Health and Human Services**
  Website: www.healthfinder.gov

Healthfinder.gov features links to more than 6,000 government and nonprofit health information resources on hundreds of health topics, including personalized health tools such as health calculators, activity and menu planners, recipes, and online checkups.

- **Well Spouse Association**
  800-838-0879
  Website: www.wellspouse.org
  E-mail: info@wellspouse.org

Well Spouse is a national membership organization that gives support to husbands, wives, and partners of the chronically ill and/or disabled. Well Spouse has a network of support groups and also offers a newsletter for spouses.

APPENDIX B

Caregiver-Specific Websites

A variety of websites offer information and support for family caregivers. Websites with key information and support for family caregivers include:

- **AgingCare.com**
  239-594-3235
  Website: www.agingcare.com
  E-mail: editor@agingcare.com

AgingCare.com helps people who care for elderly parents find support, resources, and information, as well as offering a place to connect with other caregivers.

- **AGIS Network**
  866-511-9186
  Website: www.agis.com
  E-mail: info@agis.com

AGIS.com provides education, support, expert advice, local resources, and a community for caregivers and families of the elderly.

- **CareCentral**
  Website: www.carecentral.com

CareCentral is a personalized Web service that allows users to create a private, secure online community for loved ones during significant health events. It is a free tool.

- **CareConnection.com**
  Website: www.careconnection.com

CareConnection.com is devoted to family caregivers, with up-to-date health news, elder-care specialists, insurance help, and coping advice.

- **Caregiver.com**
  800-829-2734
  Website: www.caregiver.com
  E-mail: info@caregiver.com

Caregiver.com produces *Today's Caregiver* magazine, the first national magazine dedicated to caregivers. The website includes topic-specific newsletters and online discussion lists.

- **The Caregiver Foundation of America**
  Website: www.theCaregiverFoundation.com

The Caregiver Foundation of America provides resources and services for nearly all aspects of caregiving.

- **Caregivinghelp.org**
  773-381-6008
  Website: www.caregivinghelp.org
  E-mail: caregivinghelp@cje.net

Caregivinghelp.org is a free, interactive website that features short video and text educational modules on a variety of caregiving topics; frequently asked questions that cover the different phases of caregiving; an online community monitored by a geriatric-care specialist.

- **CarePages**
  888-852-5521
  Website: www.carepages.com

CarePages are free, private Web pages that make it easy to reach out and receive messages of support and to stay connected to family, friends, co-workers, and others. The service is available to anyone caring for a loved one, but it may be particularly helpful to those who have recently found themselves in a caregiving role.

- **Centers for Medicare & Medicaid Services (CMS)**
  Website: www.medicare.gov/caregivers

Ask Medicare will help family caregivers access and use valuable health-care information, services, and resources. This new CMS initiative features a one-stop Web page for caregivers, providing easy access to useful information about Medicare and other essential resources to help with family caregiving, including links to key partner organizations that assist caregivers and beneficiaries.

- **Disability.gov**
  Website: www.disability.gov

A federal government website providing easy access to disability-related information and resources. Included is a state and local resources map, which makes it easy to locate disability-related information in specific parts of the country.

- **Family Caregiver Alliance (FCA)**
  800-445-8106
  Website: www.caregiver.org

FCA is a public voice for caregivers offering, assistance through education, services, research, and advocacy.

- **The Healing Project**
  Website: www.thehealingproject.org
  E-mail: amy@thehealingproject.org

The Healing Project is dedicated to providing support, education, resources, and help to those who face life-threatening and life-altering diseases.

- **Home Instead—Caregiverstress**
  Website: www.caregiverstress.com

Home Instead Senior Care provides information to help family caregivers find ways to cope with caregiver stress.

- **ITN Men's Caregiver Support Group program**
  Website: http://mlberg.spaces.live.com
  E-mail: mlberg.caregiver.blog@gmail.com

ITN was created as a step-by-step guide for men to develop a caregiver support group within their own communities.

- **Lotsa Helping Hands**
  Website: www.nfca.lotsahelpinghands.com
  E-mail: info@lotsahelpinghands.com

It's an easy-to-use, private group calendar, specifically designed for organizing helpers.

- **National Family Caregivers Association (NFCA)**
  800-896-3650
  Website: www.thefamilycaregiver.org

NFCA is a national nonprofit organization dedicated to empowering family caregivers to act on behalf of themselves and their loved ones, and to remove barriers to their health and well-being.

- **The National Resource Directory**
  Website: www.nationalresourcedirectory.org

Developed by the departments of Defense, Labor, and Veterans Affairs for wounded, ill and injured service members, veterans and their families, families of the fallen, and those who support them. The directory provides over 10,000 services and resources, available through governmental and non-governmental organizations, to support recovery, rehabilitation, and reintegration into the community.

- **New Health Partnerships**
  Website: www.newhealthpartnerships.org

New Health Partnerships (NHP), a program of the Institute for Healthcare Improvement, is spreading collaborative self-management support, a system of care that promotes patient/family caregiver/provider partnerships to transform care for the chronically ill. The site offers valuable tools and resources that can be easily downloaded by patients, family caregivers, and their health-care team

- **Next Step in Care**
  Website: www.nextstepincare.org

This website offers a range of guides and checklists, most intended for family caregivers of persons with serious illness, with some specifically for health-care providers. It is designed to make patients' transitions between care settings, such as rehab to home, or home to hospital, smoother and safer.

- **ShareTheCaregiving (Share the Care)**
  212-991-9688
  Website: www.sharethecare.org
  E-mail: info@sharethecare.org

ShareTheCaregiving, Inc., is a grassroots organization dedicated to preventing "caregiver burnout by promoting and educating people about the benefits of group caregiving, using the SHARE THE CARE model."

- **Strength for Caring**
  866-466-3458
  Website: www.strengthforcaring.com

Strength for Caring is an online resource and community for family caregivers that helps family caregivers take care of their loved ones and themselves. Strength for Caring is part of the Caregiver Initiative, created by Johnson & Johnson Consumer Products Company, Division of Johnson & Johnson Consumer Companies, Inc.

- **ThisCaringHome.org**
  Website: www.thiscaringhome.org

ThisCaringHome.org was produced by Weill Cornell Medical College and is a multimedia website created to provide best practices for dementia care. This website includes a "home safety virtual care" section that allows visitors to explore research-based solutions to home safety and daily care issues for people with dementia.

- **Video Caregiving**
  Website: www.videocaregiving.org

This site—a visual education tool for family caregivers of loved ones with Alzheimer's disease, strokes, or other physical disabilities—features exclusive documentary-style videos, created by a team of award-winning film producers, which follow real-life people as real-life stories and issues unfold.

- **AARP**
  800-424-3410
  Website: www.aarp.org

AARP supplies information about caregiving, long-term care, and aging, including publications and audio-visual aids for caregivers.

- **AGIS Network**
  866-511-9186
  Website: www.agis.com/
  E-mail: info@agis.com

AGIS.com provides education, support, expert advice, local resources, and a vibrant community for caregivers and families of the elderly.

- **Eldercare Locator**
  National Association of Area Agencies on Aging
  800-677-1116
  Website: www.n4a.org or www.eldercare.gov

Eldercare Locator provides referrals to area agencies on aging via ZIP code locations. Family caregivers can also find information about many eldercare issues and services available in local communities.

- **Home Instead—40/70 Rule**
  Website: www.4070talk.com

This website offers advice designed to help adult children and their aging parents deal with sensitive topics that often make conversations difficult.

- **The National Association of Professional Geriatric Care Managers**
  520-881-8008
  Website: www.caremanager.org

Geriatric care managers (GCMs) are health-care professionals, most often social workers, who help families deal with the problems and challenges associated with caring for the elderly. This national organization will refer family caregivers to their state chapters, which in turn can provide the names of GCMs in your area. This information is also available online.

- **U.S. Administration on Aging**
  202-619-0724
  Website: www.aoa.gov

The Administration on Aging is the official federal agency dedicated to the delivery of supportive home and community-based services to older individuals and their caregivers. The AoA website has a special section on family caregiving.

APPENDIX C

End-of-Life Planning, Hospice, and Bereavement Information

- **Aging with Dignity**
  888-5-WISHES (594-7437)
  Website: www.agingwithdignity.org

Aging with Dignity publishes the Five Wishes Living Will document, a very user-friendly and comprehensive document that meets legal requirements in thirty-five states.

- **Caring Connections**
  Website: www.caringinfo.org

Caring Connections provides free brochures on end-of-life topics, including advance care planning, caregiving, hospice and palliative care, pain, grief and loss, and financial issues. Caring Connections also provides advanced directives for all states.

- **HospiceDirectory.org**
  800-868-5171
  Website: http://hospicedirectory.org

This online consumer database lists hospices in North America and the U.S. All hospices are listed at no cost. It is a free service that assists families and individuals in quickly locating a hospice within their community. Also provides reliable information about hospice and end-of-life care to consumers.

- **Hospice Foundation of America**
  800-854-3402
  Website: www.hospicefoundation.org

The National Hospice Foundation hosts an annual teleconference on issues of bereavement and has publications on grief and bereavement.

- **The Compassionate Friends**
  877-969-0010
  Website: www.compassionatefriends.org

This group offers telephone support and understanding to families who have lost a child. They maintain a resource library and have a national chapter network and newsletter.

- **U.S. Department of Health and Human Services**
  National Clearinghouse for Long-Term Care Information
  Website: www.longtermcare.gov
  E-mail: aoainfo@aoa.hhs.gov

The National Clearinghouse for Long-Term Care Information provides information on planning and financing long-term care, including planning for end-of-life care and all major types of public and private financing to help cover long-term care costs.

APPENDIX D

Health Insurance Information

Family caregivers can contact their county or state Department of Health and Human Services for financial programs that may provide assistance for acquiring health insurance and prescription medications. Other possible financial resources may include social service agencies, such as Catholic Charities, the Association of Jewish Families, and children's agencies. Local chapters of voluntary health agencies may also offer financial support programs and/or information on how to apply for such programs.

- **AGIS Network**
  866-511-9186
  Website: www.agis.com/
  E-mail: info@agis.com

AGIS.com provides education, support, expert advice, local resources, and a vibrant community for caregivers and families of the elderly.

- **Benefits Check-Up and Benefits Check-Up RX**
  Website: www.benefitscheckup.org

A service of the National Council on the Aging, Benefits Check-Up and Benefits Check-Up RX help people over the age of fifty-five find federal, state, and local public and private programs that may pay for some of their medical care and/or prescription costs.

- **HealthInsurance.com**
  800-942-9019
  Website: www.healthinsurance.com

This website provides consumers and small businesses with quotes for health insurance and may help those who have lost their health insurance find an affordable alternative.

- **Medicare**
  Website: www.medicare.gov
  800-MEDICARE (633-4227)

This is the official website for the Centers for Medicare and Medicaid Services (CMS), the agency responsible for Medicare Rx.

- **Medicare Rights Center**
  888-HMO-9050
  Website: www.medicarerights.org

This is an independent source of health-care information and assistance for older and disabled Americans, their caregivers, and the professionals who serve them. Medicare Interactive (MI) is the one-stop source for information about health-care rights, options, and benefits, and it is designed to help people find answers to all their Medicare questions. The website also has a list of phone numbers for each state's State Health Insurance Assistance Program.

- **Medicare Rx Matters**
  Website: www.MedicareRxMatters.org

Designed to help users make decisions about the new Medicare prescription drug plan, this site has three specific portals: one for family caregivers, one for people with Medicare, and one for professionals. The website provides an overview, easy-to-understand steps, and information to assist users in making personal decisions about Medicare prescription drug coverage.

- **Medicine Program**
  573-996-7300
  Website: www.themedicineprogram.com

This program is for persons who do not have coverage, through insurance or government subsidies, for outpatient prescription drugs and for those who cannot afford to purchase medications at retail prices.

- **RxCompare**
  Website: www.maprx.info
  E-mail: info@maprx.info

RxCompare is a free tool developed by Medicare Access for Patients–Rx (MAPRx) to help users determine if they need to enroll in a Medicare drug plan and, if they do, to systematically compare the drug plans where they live and select the best option for their prescription needs. RxCompare works in tandem with Medicare's online prescription resource.

APPENDIX E

Homecare Agencies

- **National Association for Home Care and Hospice**
  202-547-7424
  Website: www.nahc.org

This organization for home health-care agency providers allows family caregivers to use the Internet to access a list of member agencies across the country.

- **Visiting Nurse Associations of America**
  617-737-3200
  Website: www.vnaa.org
  E-mail: vnaa@vnaa.org

VNAA promotes community-based home health care. Family caregivers can contact them to find their local VNAA.

Assisted Living, Nursing Home, and Residential Care

- **Consumer Consortium on Assisted Living (CCAL)**
  703-533-8121
  Website: www.ccal.org

CCAL is a national consumer-focused organization that is dedicated to representing the needs of residents in assisted-living facilities and to educating consumers, professionals, and the general public about assisted living issues. Family caregivers can request the publication "Choosing an Assisted Living Facility: Strategies for Making the Right Decision," which provides helpful information and a concise checklist for those contemplating this next step.

- **National Citizens' Coalition for Nursing Home Reform**
  202-332-2275
  Website: www.nccnhr.org

This organization serves as an information clearinghouse and offers referrals nationwide for help with concerns about long-term care facilities.

- **NFCA Senior Housing Locator**
  206-575-0728
  Website: www.snapforseniors.com/
  E-mail: info@snapforseniors.com

NFCA Senior Housing Locator, powered by SNAPforSeniors, is a current, comprehensive, and objective resource of senior housing in the United States. Users can also search and screen for Medicare-certified home health-care providers in their area. Download checklists and tools to help assess senior housing and care options. Exchange ideas and join discussions by participating in groups.

APPENDIX F

Respite Resources

- **Easter Seals**
  800-221-6827
  Website: http://www.easter-seals.org

Easter Seals provides a variety of services at 400 sites nationwide for children and adults with disabilities, including adult day care, in-home care, camps for special-needs children and more. Services vary by site.

- **Faith in Action**
  877-324-8411
  Website: www.fiavolunteers.org
  E-mail: info@fiavolunteers.org

Faith in Action is an interfaith volunteer caregiving program of the Robert Wood Johnson Foundation. Faith in Action makes grants to local groups, representing many faiths, who volunteer to work together to care for their neighbors who have long-term health needs. There are nearly 1,000 interfaith volunteer caregiving programs across the country.

- **Family Friends**
  National Council on the Aging, Inc.
  202-479-6672
  Website: www.family-friends.org

This group provides respite (and other services) by matching men and women volunteers over the age of fifty with families of children who have disabilities or chronic illness. Programs are located throughout the country.

- **National Adult Day Services Association, Inc.**
  866-890-7357
  Website: www.nadsa.org

This association provides information about locating adult day care centers in your local area.

- **National Respite Coalition (NRC)**
  703-256-9578
  Website: www.archrespite.org/NRC.htm

NRC provides a list of states that have respite coalitions. These state coalitions then list respite services available in their state. The majority of the information is focused on helping families of children with special needs, but lately there has been an effort to enlarge their referral base to include lifespan respite information. The NRC is working to gain passage of national lifespan respite legislation.

- **National Respite Locator Service**
  800-473-1727, ext. 222
  Website: www.respitelocator.org/index.htm

Access a list of sites nationwide. While the vast majority focus on respite care for families of special-needs children, the service now assists programs that provide respite for caregivers of adults and the elderly.

- **Shepherd's Centers of America**
  Website: www.shepherdcenters.org
  E-mail: staff@shepherdcenters.org

The organization provides respite care, telephone visitors, in-home visitors, nursing home visitors, home health aides, support groups, adult day care, and information and referrals for accessing other services available in the community. Services vary by center.

APPENDIX G

Training for Family Caregivers

Community-based resources may offer training and classes for family caregivers. Such resources may include your local hospital, home care agencies, Area Agency on Aging, voluntary health agencies, and county and state Departments of Health.

- **American Red Cross**
  202-303-4498
  Website: www.redcross.org

American Red Cross has developed training programs for family caregivers. You will need to check with your local chapter to find out if there are classes in your area.

- **National Family Caregivers Association**
  800-896-3650
  Website: www.thefamilycaregiver.org
  E-mail: info@thefamilycaregiver.org

NFCA has developed an educational workshop to teach family caregivers to communicate more effectively with health-care professionals. Check out the NFCA website to find out if there are workshops scheduled in your community.

APPENDIX H

Disease-Specific Agencies and Websites

- **Alzheimer's Association**
  Toll-free: 800-272-3900
  Website: www.alz.org

- **American Autoimmune Related Diseases Association**
  Toll-free: 800-598-4668
  Website: www.aarda.org

- **American Cancer Society**
  Toll-free: 800-ACS-2345
  Website: www.cancer.org

- **American Diabetes Association**
  Toll-free patient information: 800-342-2383
  Website: www.diabetes.org

- **American Foundation for AIDS Research**
  Toll-free: 800-39-AMFAR (392-6327)
  Website: www.amfar.org

- **American Heart Association**
  Toll-free: 800-AHA-USA1 (242-8721)
  Website: www.americanheart.org

- **American Kidney Fund**
  Toll-free Help Line: 800-638-8299
  Website: www.kidneyfund.org or www.akfinc.org

- **American Liver Foundation**
  Toll-free: 800-GO-LIVER (465-4837) or 888-4HEP-USA
  (443-7872)
  Website: www.liverfoundation.org

- **American Lung Association**
  Toll-free number to connect to local
  American Lung Association offices: 800-LUNG-USA
  Website: www.lungusa.org

- **American Pain Foundation**
  Toll-free: 888-615-PAIN (7246)
  Website: www.painfoundation.org/

- **American Parkinson Disease Association**
  800-223-2732
  Website: www.apdaparkinson.org

- **American Stroke Association**
  Toll-Free: 888-4-STROKE (478-7653)
  Website: www.strokeassociation.org

- **American Tinnitus Association**
  Toll-free: 800-634-8978
  Website: www.ata.org

- **ALS Association**
  Toll-free: 800-782-4747
  Website: www.alsa.org

- **Arthritis Foundation**
  Toll-free 800-283-7800
  Website: www.arthritis.org

- **Asthma & Allergy Foundation of America**
  Toll-free: 800-7-ASTHMA
  Website: www.aafa.org

- **Cancer and Careers**
  Website: www.cancerandcareers.org

Cancer and Careers is committed to changing the face of cancer in the workplace by providing a comprehensive website, free publications, and a series of support groups and educational seminars for employees with cancer.

- **Cancer Financial Assistance Coalition**
  Website: www.cancerfac.org
  Phone: 800-813-HOPE (813-4673)

CancerCare is a member of the coalition. Search the website by location or diagnosis to find organizations that provide financial help for your specific situation.

- **Cancer Research and Prevention Foundation**
  Toll-free: 800-227-CRFA (227-2732)
  Website: www.preventcancer.org

- **Crohn's & Colitis Foundation of America**
  Toll-free: 800-343-3637 (to order brochures and for general information)
  Website: www.ccfa.org

- **Cystic Fibrosis Foundation**
  800-FIGHT CF (344-4823)
  Website: www.cff.org

- **Easter Seals**
  Toll-free: 800-221-6827
  Website: www.easter-seals.org

- **Epilepsy Foundation**
  Toll Free: 800-332-1000
  Website: www.epilepsyfoundation.org

- **The Foundation Fighting Blindness**
  Toll-free: 888-394-3937
  Website: www.blindness.org

- **Huntington's Disease Society of America**
  Toll-free: 800-345-HDSA
  Website: www.hdsa.org

- **Kidney Cancer Association**
  Toll-free: 800-850-9132
  Website: www.kidneycancerassociation.org

- **The Leukemia & Lymphoma Society**
  Toll-free: 800-955-4572
  Website: www.leukemia-lymphoma.org

- **Lupus Foundation of America**
  Toll-free information request line: 800-558-0121
  Website: www.lupus.org

- **March of Dimes Birth Defects Foundation**
  March of Dimes Resource Center
  Toll-free: 888-663-4637
  Website: www.modimes.org

- **Michael J. Fox Foundation for Parkinson's Research**
  Toll-free at 1-800-708-7644
  Website: www.michaeljfox.org

- **Muhammad Ali Parkinson Center**
  602-406-4931
  Website: www.maprc.com

- **Myasthenia Gravis Foundation of America**
  Toll-free: 800-541-5454
  Website: www.myasthenia.org

- **Myositis Association**
  Toll-free: 800-821-7356
  Website: www.myositis.org

- **National Down Syndrome Society**
  Toll-free: 800-221-4602
  Website: www.ndss.org

- **National Hemophilia Foundation**
  Toll-free: 800-42-HANDI (424-2634)
  Website: www.hemophilia.org

- **National Mental Health Association**
  Toll Free: 800-969-NMHA (6642)
  Website: www.nmha.org

- **National Multiple Sclerosis Society**
  Toll-free: 800-FIGHT-MS (344-4867)
  Website: www.nationalmssociety.org or www.nmss.org

- **National Organization for Rare Disorders**
  800-999-6673
  Website: www.rarediseases.org

- **National Osteoporosis Foundation**
  202-223-2226
  Website: www.nof.org

- **National Parkinson Foundation, Inc.**
  800-327-4545
  Website: www.parkinson.org

- **National Psoriasis Foundation**
  Toll-free: 800-723-9166
  Website: www.psoriasis.org

- **National Sleep Foundation**
  202-347-3471
  Website: www.sleepfoundation.org

- **Osteogenesis Imperfecta Foundation**
  Toll-free: 800-981-BONE (2663)
  Website: www.oif.org

- **The Paget Foundation**
  Toll-free: 800-23-PAGET (237-2438)
  Website: www.paget.org

- **Parkinson's Disease Foundation**
  (212) 923-4700
  Website: www.pdf.org

- **Partners Against Pain**
  888-726-7535
  Website: www.partnersagainstpain.com

- **Sjogren's Syndrome Foundation**
  Toll-Free: 800-475-6473
  Website: www.sjogrens.org

- **Spina Bifida Association of America**
  Toll-free: 800-621-3141
  Website: www.sbaa.org

- **Tourette Syndrome Association, Inc.**
  Toll-free: 888-4-TOURET (486-8738)
  Website: www.tsa-usa.org

- **United Ostomy Association**
  Toll-free: 800-826-0826
  Website: www.uoaa.org

- **United Cerebral Palsy**
  800-872-5827
  Website: www.ucp.org

APPENDIX I

Adaptive Equipment Resources

Adaptive equipment is available to assist in all aspects of daily living, including grooming, bathing, eating, writing, and mobility. The adaptive devices mentioned in chapter five (and many more not mentioned) can be ordered from the following websites. The websites presented below are not all-inclusive. You can perform a search with keywords "adaptive equipment" to get a more comprehensive listing of vendors.

www.arthritissupplies.com
www.caregiverproducts.com
www.mobility-Aids.com
www.wrightstuff.com
www.ncmedical.com
www.sammonspreston.com

APPENDIX J

Home Assessment Checklist

HOME ENTRY

PROBLEM	SOLUTION
☐ Unable to safely negotiate stairs.	☐ Add ramp
☐ Risers are too high.	☐ Add rails
☐ Nosings catch on foot. (Nosings are extensions or lips that extend past the riser of the step)	☐ Bevel nosing
	☐ Close risers
	☐ Use non-slip treads: stairs/ramp
☐ Open riser catches foot	☐ Use chair lift
☐ Slips on stairs	☐ Mark edge of each tread with distinguishing strip
☐ Needs balance support	
☐ Difficulty distinguishing edges or thresholds	☐ Change ramp slope
	☐ Increase lighting

NOTES

DOORS

PROBLEM	SOLUTION
☐ Too narrow for passage	☐ Use swing-clear hinges (adds 1½ to 1¾ inches to the thickness of the door)
☐ Landing too small to manage door with wheelchair or assistive device	☐ Remove door stops (adds ¾ inch)
☐ Thresholds—tripping hazard or a barrier	☐ Remove door
☐ Door mats—tripping hazard	☐ Use automatic door opener
☐ Difficulty managing door handle	☐ Enlarge landing
☐ Difficulty managing lock	☐ Remove threshold
☐ Door swing hazard (interior door)	☐ Change threshold to lower profile

NOTES	SOLUTION (cont.)
	☐ Bevel ramp for threshold
	☐ Replace door
	☐ sliding
	☐ folding
	☐ pocket
	☐ swing (widen)
	☐ Secure doormat
	☐ Recess to be flush
	☐ Add kick-plates
	☐ Install lever adapter for cylinder knob
	☐ Install lever hardware (doorknob)
	☐ Install loop hardware (doorknob)
	☐ Use slide bolts
	☐ Relocate lock
	☐ Install vision panels

BATHROOM

PROBLEM	SOLUTION

☐ Sink
  ☐ No clearance beneath for wheelchair
  ☐ Too low—bending difficulty
  ☐ Limited hand dexterity
☐ Toilets
  ☐ Seat height too high
  ☐ Seat height too low
  ☐ Difficulty with toilet transfer
☐ Shower/Tub
  ☐ Transfer to tub unsafe
  ☐ Inability to stand
  ☐ Decreased balance in tub
	☐ Remove sink cabinet doors
	  ☐ cover pipes (insulation)
	  ☐ add decorative curtains
	☐ Remove cabinet wall mounts
	  ☐ cover pipes (insulation)
	  ☐ add decorative curtains
	☐ Raise sink/vanity
	☐ Lower sink/vanity
	☐ Replace knobs with single-lever faucet
	☐ Replace knobs with double-levers or cross knobs

NOTES	☐ Raise toilet seat
	☐ Use foot stool
	☐ Install grab-bars
	☐ wall mount
	☐ sheltering arms
	☐ pivoting
	☐ Install tub seat
	☐ Install tub transfer bench
	☐ Install tub chair
	☐ Use handheld shower
	☐ Use tub lifts
	☐ Add non-skid surface

	☐ Add wall mount grab-bars
	☐ Add removable tub grab-bars
	☐ Add roll-in shower
	☐ Use shower chair
	☐ Use anti-scald temperature controls
	☐ Install emergency call button or telephone, or make sure the nearest existing telephone can be safely brought into bathroom
	☐ Make sure mirror and medicine cabinet are easy to use; bottom edge of mirror should be no higher than 42 inches from floor. Install tilting mirror
	☐ Install heat lamp
	☐ Install ceiling vent fan

KITCHEN

PROBLEM	SOLUTION
☐ Difficulty accessing freezer	☐ Use a side-by-side refrigerator/freezer
☐ Counter/work surface	
☐ too high	☐ Use a stand-alone table
☐ too low	☐ Use wheelchair lap board
☐ no wheelchair clearance underneath	☐ Install folding/pull-out shelves
☐ impaired hand dexterity	☐ Use wood boards across drawers
☐ Sink	☐ Remove base cabinets
☐ too deep	☐ Remove cabinet drawers
☐ no clearance beneath for wheelchair	☐ Use spiked cutting boards
☐ Cooktop	☐ Replace/add counters; locate according to specific needs
☐ wheelchair user cannot reach back burners	☐ adjustable
☐ difficult visibility to cook	☐ manual
☐ difficulty moving pots and pans full of water or food	☐ electric
☐ Cooktop	☐ Add "hot item" shelf to or next to oven
☐ wheelchair user cannot reach back burners	☐ Install rack
☐ difficult visibility to cook	☐ Remove cabinet doors
☐ difficulty moving pots and pans full of water or food	☐ Remove cabinet/wall mount sink
☐ Storage/cabinets	☐ Use handheld hose/sprayer
	☐ Use staggered burners
	☐ Add mirror above stove
	☐ Use flush ceramic cooktops
	☐ Add wall mount over microwave
	Replace storage drawer hardware with easy-gliding hardware or simplify

NOTES

☐ current operations; include C- or D-shaped handles

☐ Install lazy Susan in corner cabinetry

☐ Consider open or pull-out shelves (open shelves above counter provide better storage for older care-receivers, especially if kept as low as possible); if not open shelves, consider transparent front for easy visibility to the inside

☐ Add towel rack, low shelves to cabinet doors

☐ Use electric can opener, jar cover opener, grip enhancer, timer with large numbers, long-handle "reacher"

FLOORS

PROBLEM	SOLUTION
☐ Slipping, tripping, falling	☐ Secure rug corners and edges; area rugs can help define areas
NOTES	☐ Cover potentially slippery floors with textured runners, carpet
	☐ Use vinyl, rubber, cork floor tile
	☐ Use non-glare material
	☐ Use heavyweight, high-density, short pile level carpet

LIGHTING

PROBLEM	SOLUTION
☐ Slipping, tripping, falling	☐ Install fixtures at locations that care-receiver uses most often, or place lamps adjacent to most-used locations
NOTES	☐ Use light fixtures with more than one bulb; increase light bulb wattage
	☐ Add light switches at door to each room
	☐ Use larger rocker switches
	☐ Locate switches and thermostats no higher than 48 inches above floor (specific location depending on needs)
	☐ Paint light switches a contrasting color to wall
	☐ Put locator lights on switches
	☐ Add a strobe light on doorbell
	☐ Use light dimmer switches
	☐ Install stair light
	☐ Use blinds or shades to control glare from outdoor light
	☐ Paint walls a light color; these tend to give off more light.
	☐ If glare is a problem, use textured wall paper or matte paint on walls
	☐ Use color to define an area or to heighten contrast between objects or areas, including where the wall meets the floor
	☐ Locate electric outlets higher than standard height; ideally, at least 27 inches from the floor

STORAGE

PROBLEM	SOLUTION
☐ Cannot access tools or personal items	☐ Use track sliding doors (possibly tracks on top and bottom); bi-fold doors are also easy to use
NOTES	☐ Use roll-out drawers or other drawers with easy-to-use-hardware
	☐ Use dual height clothes rails or adjustable rods (possibly a rotating carousel)
	☐ Rearrange storage for maximum usefulness, given potential reaching, stretching, and bending limitations

ABOUT THE AUTHOR

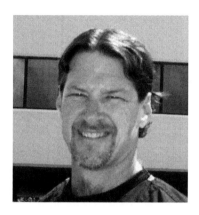

Kevin Lockette has been a practicing physical therapist in the rehabilitation field since 1989 and is co-owner—with his wife,
Ginger—of Ohana Pacific Rehab Services (www.ohanapacificre-
hab.com), LLC, in Honolulu, Hawaii. He is the primary author of a
landmark medical text on rehabilitation, *Conditioning with Physical
Disabilities* (Human Kinetic Publishers, 1994). He recently au-
thored *Move It—An Exercise and Mobility Guide for People with
Parkinson's Disease* (www.parkinsonsmoveit.com) and has written
numerous articles and lectured extensively in the area of exercise,
with emphasis on physical disabilities.

Kevin is a past head coach for the United States Disabled Sports
Team (a member of the U.S. Olympic Committee) and coached
in international games, including the World Championships and
the Paralympics in Barcelona, Spain, in 1992. Presently, Kevin
serves on the board of directors for the Hawaii Parkinson Disease
Association, Clinical Advisory Counsel for the Hawaii chapter of

the MS Society and is co-chairman of the state of Hawaii's Fall Prevention Consortium.

Kevin enjoys canoe-paddling and weight-lifting. He is an avid college basketball fan and attends University of Hawaii sports whenever he can. Kevin is the father of a daughter and son (Griffin and Hudson, respectively), as well as being an athlete and history buff. He plays harmonica and ukulele and has a love for the blues.